KT-151-947

# thefacts

# Chronic fatigue syndrome (CFS/ME)

SECOND EDITION

## FRANKIE CAMPLING

A person with CFS/ME

## MICHAEL SHARPE

Professor of Psychological Medicine and
Symptom Research, University of Edinburgh,
Scotland, UK

OXFORD
UNIVERSITY PRESS

# OXFORD
UNIVERSITY PRESS

Great Clarendon Street, Oxford OX2 6DP

Oxford University Press is a department of the University of Oxford.
It furthers the University's objective of excellence in research, scholarship,
and education by publishing worldwide in

Oxford New York

Auckland Cape Town Dar es Salaam Hong Kong Karachi
Kuala Lumpur Madrid Melbourne Mexico City Nairobi
New Delhi Shanghai Taipei Toronto

With offices in

Argentina Austria Brazil Chile Czech Republic France Greece
Guatemala Hungary Italy Japan Poland Portugal Singapore
South Korea Switzerland Thailand Turkey Ukraine Vietnam

Oxford is a registered trade mark of Oxford University Press
in the UK and in certain other countries

Published in the United States
by Oxford University Press Inc., New York

British Library Cataloguing in Publication Data

Data available

Library of Congress Cataloging in Publication Data

Campling, Frankie.
  Chronic fatigue syndrome (CFS/ME) / Frankie Campling,
  Michael Sharpe. – 2nd ed.
  p. cm. – (the facts)
  Includes index.
  ISBN–13: 978–0–19–923316–8
1. Chronic fatigue syndrome–Popular Works. I. Sharpe, Michael. II. Title.
  RB150. F37C36 2008
  616′. 0478–dc22

                                                                          2008016322

Typeset by Cepha Imaging Pvt. Ltd., Bangalore, India
Printed in Great Britain
on acid-free paper by
Ashford Colour Press Ltd, Gosport, Hampshire

ISBN 978–0–19–923316–8

3 5 7 9 10 8 6 4

# Forewords

CFS/ME, chronic fatigue syndrome, or myalgic encephalomyelitis—as it can be mundanely or scarily known—is a common, beastly, variable, confusing, invisible, and pervasive illness. It profoundly changes just about everything in the life of an affected person, as well as in those around them. The body sends out multiple confusing distress signals (symptoms), the 'little grey cells' don't seem to work properly ('brain fog'), simple things become complicated, normal activities and roles are hard to sustain, confidence fails, and other people seem to react differently.

CFS/ME seems especially liable to elicit controversy and polarized views from those who do, and those who don't, know about it. Despite its enormous personal and social impact, and despite being around for centuries, it is one of the most under-researched areas of clinical medicine, although happily that is changing. Indeed, lack of knowledge is part of the reason for controversy, because people tend to fill the gaps in understanding with strong opinions!

This illness doesn't readily fit some prevailing medical or social paradigms. This leads some people to diminish, deny, or even neglect those affected. Perhaps this is an unconscious defence against ignorance and the threat of something that challenges our assumptions about the world. Meanwhile, people with CFS/ME feel increasingly alienated, both from themselves and from others, doubling the burden of illness.

Patients, and those close to them, need a map and a compass when landed in this unexpected and hostile terrain. So it is a joy to welcome the new edition of this outstanding book on CFS/ME. As before, it presents a straightforward, commonsense approach, supported by the twin pillars of patient experience and research evidence. As Campling and Sharpe emphasise, despite the gaps in knowledge, we do actually know a lot about how to recognize and manage this illness. And they set it out with great clarity.

As an experienced clinician in this field, I have heard so many stories about the things that people find difficult or even counter-intuitive in this illness.

This book explains them all, with a light and gentle style that is very refreshing. I have to confess that my first peep was to check that they still had my favourite chapter: 'What gets in the way of being sensible?'. But you can't read or understand that until you have read most of the rest!

If you have the illness, this can be your companion and guide; when you think you are lost, you can find your way again. When people around you don't seem to understand, just make sure they know this is the 'manual'; they may peep at it, when you are not looking! If you look after people affected, personally or professionally, this is a great place to start; and to revisit regularly.

CFS/ME is an unfamiliar and frightening place to be. But with this map and compass, you will find your way, you may rediscover yourself, and you can make the unexpected journey your own again.

Professor Anthony J Pinching
Associate Dean for Cornwall, Peninsula Medical School

Whilst we usually think of treatments as pills, books can also be effective therapies. In *Chronic Fatigue Syndrome (CFS/ME): The Facts*, Frankie Campling and Michael Sharpe have written an extremely therapeutic book.

In my role as an educator and as a clinician working in a CFS/ME clinic, I have frequently recommended this book to both patients and to colleagues. Patients have found it clear, authoritative, and helpful, while practitioners, many of whom feel ill-equipped to manage patients with CFS/ME, are grateful for a clear jargon-free account of the condition, based firmly on research evidence, which they can firmly recommend to patients and carers.

Peter D Campion
Emeritus Professor of Primary Care Medicine, University of Hull.

# Contents

Section three

## Special issues

Appendices

# Introduction

This book is aimed primarily at people suffering from chronic fatigue ayndrome (CFS/ME), their carers, families, and friends, though we hope that other people who want to understand more about this illness may also read it. We want to say, right from the start, that we believe that people suffering from CFS/ME have a genuine, distressing, and debilitating illness. We also believe that that there is much that can be done to help.

We both have wide experience of the illness going back 15 years and more— Frankie Campling as a person with CFS/ME who has done telephone support work for others like herself, and Michael Sharpe as a clinician and researcher who has run specialist clinical services for CFS/ME and published widely on the illness. Our combined experience enables us to see the illness from the perspectives of both medical science and sufferers. We hope that this collaboration of doctor and patient will offer our readers a unique perspective on CFS/ME, on what doctors can do to help, and especially what sufferers can do to help themselves.

Our main aims in writing this book were:

- to explain what is meant by CFS/ME and how it is diagnosed
- to provide research-based information on possible causes and treatments
- to help our readers evaluate new findings and claims about CFS/ME
- to help patients and carers make informed decisions about treatment
- to offer practical guidance on what patients can do to help themselves.

We know that many people with CFS/ME suffer greatly because some of those around them (though definitely **not** us) do not believe that they are ill or even suggest the illness is imaginary or 'all in the mind'. We talk about this later, suggesting why this disbelief occurs, reviewing evidence that indicates that CFS/ME is a 'real' illness, and suggesting ways of communicating with family, friends, and doctors that will minimize this most distressing problem.

When reading this book you may be surprised or even somewhat disconcerted to find that we spend a good deal of time discussing behavioural and psychological strategies and rather less on drug treatments. This is because both the available research evidence and our own experience show that such strategies are the most helpful treatments. Drug therapy has a role, but the evidence for its effectiveness is less good. As with all illnesses, the way sufferers cope will influence both their quality of life and the outcome of the illness. Along with a number of other illnesses, the fact that we do not yet fully understand the causes of CFS/ME does not mean that we are unable work out how best to manage it. This new edition of the book has given us a welcome opportunity to include the latest information on research and treatment. We hope you will find this helpful.

We should stress that though we can offer you a 'map' of scientific information about CFS/ME and its treatment, you as a patient are the expert on the 'territory' of your own illness. We can offer you advice about management strategies that other patients have found helpful, but you are the one to choose whether or not to try them. If you do make this choice, we can be tour guides, but you are the one who will have to do the walking. All we ask is that you should approach what we write with an open mind. We very much hope that you will want to try out the techniques we suggest. We also hope that you will find, as others have, that they will improve your situation and that, even if they do not produce a cure, they will give you a sense of greater control over the illness and hope for the future.

One of the most important of the management strategies we discuss is that of pacing yourself carefully, always stopping before you get too tired. We suggest that you read this book in a similar way. Take it slowly. Do not try to read it all in one sitting. You will probably get more out of it if you read a chapter or two and then stop for a rest. We have tried to keep our language simple, but are aware that you may still come across unfamiliar medical words and so have included a glossary of such words at the back of the book.

In conclusion, we hope that that you will find this book helpful and that it will improve your understanding of CFS/ME. We also hope that it will give you ideas about what **you** can do to improve both your state of health and your quality of life.

# Acknowledgements

We are very grateful to those people, both clinicians and patients, who read the manuscript and gave us such valuable comments and suggestions. These include Hilary Briars, Dr John Campling, Dr Zoe Dunhill, Dr Birgitta Evengard, Dr William Hamilton, Katherine Kephalas, Dr Ivana Klimes, Dr Andrew Lloyd, Dr Duncan Manders, Dr Peter White, and Dr David Wilks, though many others have given us really helpful assistance.

Most of all though, we want to thank all the people with CFS/ME whom we have worked with over the last 15 and more years. They have taught us so much about what suffering from CFS/ME is like and what they have found helpful. This book is dedicated to them.

# Chronic fatigue syndrome (CFS/ME): its nature, diagnosis, and treatment

# 1

# Our aims in this section

## ⊃ Key points

◆ There are many questions asked about CFS/ME but few facts

◆ Facts are those answers supported by sound scientific research; answers based only on clinical experience or anecdote may be the best we have, but they are not facts

◆ The symptoms of CFS/ME are real, even if medical tests are normal

## The questions that get asked

If you or someone you know has been diagnosed as having chronic fatigue syndrome or myalgic encephalomyelitis (CFS/ME) you are likely to have a lot of questions you want answered. During the 15 years and more that we have been working with those suffering from this illness, we have become familiar with the questions that are the most commonly asked. These are:

◆ Is it a real illness?

◆ What should it be called and why?

◆ What is the illness?

◆ How is it diagnosed?

◆ What other conditions is it linked to?

◆ Who gets it?

◆ What is the cause?

◆ What is the best treatment?

◆ Do people get better?

In this section of the book we will review the known facts about CFS/ME to provide the best available answers to these and other questions.

# How should we decide what is a 'fact'?

The title of this book is 'Chronic fatigue syndrome (CFS/ME): the facts'. A fact is something known to be true. In science that means information that is supported by good research evidence. You may be aware that CFS/ME is an illness about which facts seem to be scarce and theories plentiful. We have tried to marshal the facts and, when there are no facts to offer, the best information and advice we can. We have done this because we believe that moving forward with scepticism is better than being paralysed by uncertainty.

In the chapters that follow we will indicate which statements are facts, which are informed opinion, and which are merely ideas and anecdote by pointing out the quality of evidence supporting them. We have distinguished three different types of evidence:

◆ *Sound scientific research findings.* This usually means findings from high-quality research that have been found by more than one group of researchers and which are accepted as true by most experts. These are facts.

◆ *Consistent clinical experience.* This is where there is some suggestive research evidence or where there is a degree of consensus amongst health professionals. This is informed opinion.

◆ *Anecdote.* This is the weakest evidence. It covers the area of disputed or unreplicated scientific reports and 'we have heard from some people that they have found such-and-such helpful'. These are merely ideas and anecdote.

You should bear in mind the level of evidence for everything you read about CFS/ME (including this book!). We would encourage you to be suitably sceptical where the evidence is weak.

In Appendix 3 we have included guidelines for critically evaluating information about CFS/ME (the DISCERN instrument). You might wish to practise them by applying them to this book!

# Is CFS/ME real?

One of the most difficult issues for both patients and doctors when a diagnosis of CFS/ME is made is how to understand it. What sort of an illness is it that does not show up on any tests? Some people (and that includes some doctors) believe inaccurately that normal test results mean that there is nothing wrong with the person. However, the 'normal test' problem may lead to patients feeling that their complaints have been ignored, that they have been accused of making them up, or that their problem is 'all in the mind'. To make matters worse, many people tend to regard those illnesses thought of as 'mental' as indicating that a person is weak, in some way at fault for being ill, or even malingering.

These misconceptions can be very upsetting, but they **are** misconceptions. They result from two errors. The first error is the belief that standard *medical* tests can detect all disturbances in bodily functioning. They cannot; but, as they say, 'absence of evidence does not mean evidence of absence'. However, in patients with CFS/ME and other related 'unexplained' illnesses, *research* tests can frequently detect disturbances in the functioning of the body and especially some in the nervous system.

The second error is the belief that people can be regarded as being made of two separate parts—a 'mind' and a 'body'—and a belief that if nothing can be found wrong with the body then the problem must be in the mind. This is an outmoded way of thinking about illness. A more modern view is that mind and body are not separate but rather two sides of the same coin: states of mind have parallel states of brain. Dividing illness into categories of **either** mental/psychiatric **or** physical/medical is a serious and potentially harmful mistake. Rather there are physical, psychological and social aspects of all illnesses—including CFS/ME.

# 2

# What should it be called and why?

---

> ## ➡ Key points
>
> ◆ There are many names for this illness, which can be confusing
>
> ◆ Most doctors prefer the name chronic fatigue syndrome (CFS)
>
> ◆ Many patients prefer ME (myalgic encephalomyelitis/encephalopathy) or CFIDS (chronic fatigue and immune system dysfunction syndrome)
>
> ◆ Like most recent official reports, we use the name CFS/ME

## What's in a name?

Various names are used for this illness, which can be very confusing. What are the different names, and where do they come from? Do they all mean the same thing? What name should we use? Well, to start with the first question (and ignoring the disgusting and inaccurate 'yuppie flu'), the names used for this condition can be:

### Chronic fatigue syndrome (CFS)

Chronic fatigue syndrome (CFS) is now the name most generally used by doctors and the one they mostly prefer. In medical language, 'chronic' means that an illness has been present for a long time, usually more than 6 months. 'Chronic' is distinguished from 'acute' (which means an illness of rapid and severe onset but often of short duration). A syndrome is an illness or condition that is diagnosed on the basis of a combination of symptoms and/or signs (as opposed to abnormalities on tests). In CFS, the symptom shared by all sufferers is severe fatigue. Other symptoms commonly present are muscle aches, poor concentration, and feeling unwell after exertion. (We will look at other symptoms in Chapter 3). Hence the term 'chronic fatigue syndrome' for a condition that has been present for 6 months or more and is diagnosed on the basis of symptoms of which a major one is fatigue.

## Myalgic encephalomyelitis/encephalopathy (ME)

This name is also used. It was originally given to an acute, medically unexplained illness that occurred among the staff of the Royal Free Hospital, London in the 1950s. Many doctors do not agree with applying this name to patients with chronic fatigue symptoms for two reasons. The first is that many of the symptoms of the Royal Free outbreak were different from those experienced by CFS patients today. The second is that this name is potentially misleading as, although many patients do have myalgia (this simply means muscle pain), there is no good evidence that they have encephalomyelitis (inflammation of the brain and spinal cord). An alternative term 'myalgic encephalopathy' has been suggested to avoid the implication of inflammation, but this still implies an unproven brain disease. Despite these reservations 'ME' is a name commonly used by patients, the general public, the media, and some doctors.

## Chronic fatigue and immune dysfunction syndrome (CFIDS)

Patients and some doctors in the USA use this name. It highlights not only the fatigue but also changes in the immune system. Whilst relatively small changes have been found in the functioning of the immune system in some patients (as they can be in many illnesses), it is still not clear how important these are in causing the symptoms. Furthermore, the apparent similarity with the term AIDS (acquired immune deficiency syndrome), in which there is an important and severe disturbance of immune functioning, is potentially misleading (and unnecessarily worrying).

## Post-viral fatigue syndrome (PVFS)

This label is sometimes used by doctors in cases which appeared to have started with a viral illness. 'Post-viral' simply means after a virus. It does not necessarily mean that a virus is causing the continuing condition. As viral infections are very common, it can be difficult to be certain that any viral infection was the cause or not. The term does not really mean anything different from CFS.

## Neurasthenia

This name was used in the late 1800s to describe a condition that was probably much the same thing as CFS. The term literally means 'weak nerves'.

Later on this diagnosis fell out of favour—although doctors still occasionally use it.

### Names of epidemics

Some other names refer to places where a number of patients became ill with something similar—Los Angeles and Akureyri are examples. The relationship of these apparent epidemics to the more common cases is unclear. These names are therefore best avoided in routine use.

## Why do most doctors call it 'chronic fatigue syndrome'?

The term 'chronic fatigue syndrome' was officially coined in the late 1980s. Prior to that time people suffering from severe and chronic fatigue that could not be medically explained were given a variety of diagnoses. One common diagnosis was infection with Epstein–Barr virus (EBV), the virus that causes glandular fever. Other infections blamed included chronic brucellosis (a rare infection transmitted from cows).

By the 1980s the accumulating scientific evidence showed that these infections were not the cause of the chronic fatigue in most cases. In 1988 a group of physicians met at the Centers for Disease Control (CDC) in Atlanta, USA to discuss this matter. They chose the name chronic fatigue syndrome (CFS). They chose this name because it simply described the illness (although admittedly emphasizing one symptom) and did not make any assumptions about the cause, which they agreed was unknown. Researchers in the UK and Australia also independently agreed to use this name. It was hoped that having one name that simply described the illness would make it easier to compare research findings.

## What is wrong with the name 'chronic fatigue syndrome'?

Although it has become the most commonly used name, some patients are unhappy about their illness being called chronic fatigue syndrome. Two main reasons are given for this. First, naming the illness only after a symptom and not a disease process is seen by some as implying it is not a real illness. Secondly, mentioning only fatigue is seen as failing to convey the severity of illness and range of symptoms patients with CFS may suffer and encourages comments such as 'Well we all get tired you know'.

Given these feelings, it is not surprising that there have been campaigns to have the name changed. Alternatives proposed include eponyms—using the name of someone well known who has studied the illness (such as Melvin Ramsay) or someone who apparently suffered from it (such as Florence Nightingale). Others have favoured a name that sounds more like a medical disease than CFS (such as myalgic encephalopathy—a different version of ME).

Whatever the arguments for and against CFS as a name, changing it would not be easy. It has been helpful to researchers to have an agreed name, and the term CFS has become established in medical journals and textbooks (and on most scientific databases). It would be a major task to convince doctors and researchers that more benefit than harm will result from changing it. It seems likely that any change in name will have to await a better understanding of the cause of the illness or illnesses that are currently referred to as CFS.

## So do these names all refer to the same illness?

The names in common usage today probably do all refer to much the same collection of symptoms, though they differ in their historical origins and in what they imply about the nature of the illness. However, it seems increasingly likely that patients with CFS do not all have exactly the same condition even though they may experience somewhat similar symptoms. This is what doctors mean when they talk of a 'heterogeneous' condition. In time, different subgroups may be identified.

Some people believe that there is a subgroup of patients with CFS who have a particularly severe illness (which they would prefer to be called ME), which should be researched and treated differently from CFS. This suggestion may be correct, but it has not yet been proved.

## The name we are using

Chronic fatigue syndrome (CFS) is the current medically preferred name for the illness and so we will use it. However, the term ME is also used very often to refer to the same illness (particularly by patients), so we will use the now commonly used combined term 'CFS/ME' in this book.

There are a number of different names that have been or are still being used to label this illness. In general they refer to similar if not identical conditions and so are largely interchangeable. In due course, research may allow the illness to be split into different subtypes. At present, chronic fatigue syndrome (CFS) is the name most favoured by doctors. Some patients prefer ME. In this book, we will use the combined term CFS/ME.

# 3

# What is chronic fatigue syndrome (CFS/ME)?

> ## ➡ Key points
>
> ◆ Fatigue is common and can be caused by different factors and illnesses
>
> ◆ Persistent, severe fatigue that restricts activity and is not caused by another medical condition may lead to a diagnosis of CFS
>
> ◆ Detailed definitions (criteria) for diagnosing CFS/ME have been produced for **research** purposes— they list specific symptoms not caused by another illness

## What is fatigue?

As 'fatigue' forms part of the medical name, it seems sensible to talk about that first. People often mean different things when they talk about fatigue. They may mean:

◆ a feeling of sleepiness

◆ a reluctance to start a task

◆ an inability to keep going at a task

◆ feeling terrible after exertion.

Fatigue may also refer to the normal weariness experienced after having worked hard. These varied meanings are a source of confusion. It is important when talking about fatigue to specify what sort of fatigue we mean. Certainly the fatigue experienced by people with CFS/ME is very different from 'everyday' tiredness.

# When is fatigue an illness?

Fatigue is very common. Surveys have shown that almost a quarter of the population, if asked, will say that fatigue has been a problem for them over the last month. Fatigue of some degree is normal and often related to periods of stress, overwork, depression, or loss of sleep. People usually consult a doctor about fatigue when it is both persistent and sufficiently severe to interfere with daily activities. This is when fatigue becomes a major problem for patients and clinically significant to doctors. It may then be considered as an illness.

# Types of fatiguing illness

Persistent severe fatigue can be caused by many diseases. The type of fatigue may give a clue to the nature of the disease:

♦ Fatigue that is described as an overwhelming need to fall asleep points to a sleep problem.

♦ Fatigue that feels like a loss of motivation, interest, and enjoyment (sometimes called anhedonia) suggests depression.

The typical fatigue of CFS/ME is described as a feeling of exhaustion, weariness, and debility that makes it difficult to start or persist in a physical or mental task and that is made worse by the effort of attempting it. People with CFS/ME usually say that their fatigue is very different from the tiredness they experienced before they were ill and describe it as feeling not just exhausted but 'really ill'. Persistent, severe fatigue of this type that restricts normal activity and is not explained by another condition may lead to a diagnosis of CFS/ME.

# A research definition of CFS/ME

When the name CFS was coined in 1988 it was linked to a detailed definition of the illness. In 1991 a group of British clinicians and researchers met in Oxford, UK and agreed on what are now known as the 'Oxford criteria' for CFS (criteria are standards by which something is judged). In 1994 the Centers for Disease Control (CDC) decided to revise their own case definition to produce an 'international definition'. Today the 1991 Oxford and the 1994 International CDC definitions are the currently accepted definitions for CFS. Guidance has also been published on how the 1994 criteria should be applied. In 2003 a new 'Canadian' definition was proposed. This has enjoyed some popularity as it is described in very medical terms, but it is very hard to apply in practice and is not in widespread use by doctors. In Appendix 3 we have listed the medical papers that give details of these criteria.

It is important to remember that there is nothing absolute about these criteria. They were constructed by committees (have you heard the joke that a camel is a horse designed by a committee?) and were intended to provide standard definitions for **research** studies, not for clinical practice where diagnoses may be made and used more pragmatically. They will be reviewed and it is likely at some point in the future, when our understanding of the processes that give rise to the symptoms of CFS is better, they will be superseded. For the moment they are the best we have.

The main parts of the current definitions are:

- the symptom of severe fatigue

- other specified symptoms

- a reduced level of activity

- an illness lasting at least 6 months

- no better medical explanation for the fatigue.

An extended period with the symptoms was specified in order to separate CFS from the brief fatigue states that can occur after almost any illness (although the precise figure of 6 months is arbitrary).

## What other symptoms are there?

The symptoms listed in the International CDC definition of CFS/ME are:

- malaise (feeling ill) after exertion

- difficulties with memory and concentration

- sore throat

- tender lymph nodes ('glands' in the neck, armpit, and groin)

- myalgia (muscle pain)

- arthralgia (joint pain)

- headaches

- disturbed and unrefreshing sleep.

As well as these symptoms, people with CFS/ME often experience:

- abdominal and digestive problems

- chest pains

- nausea (feeling sick)

- feeling inappropriately hot or cold

- night sweats

- looking pale when tired

- feeling dizzy or light headed

- problems with balance

- worsening of symptoms before a menstrual period

- hearing problems such as hyperacusis (painful sensitivity to noises)

- eye problems such as pain around the eyes, difficulty focusing, and sensitivity to bright lights.

Some of these symptoms can be frightening. You may fear that they indicate a life-threatening disease. If you have moments like this, do discuss your fears with your doctor. In Chapter 4 we will tell you about the routine medical tests you are likely to have had and what conditions they will have ruled out.

## How common is CFS/ME?

You may remember that earlier we mentioned surveys in which it was found that almost a quarter of the population complain of a problem with fatigue. CFS/ME is of course a good deal less common than that. Available studies suggest that it is present in between 2 people in every 1000 (0.2%) and 20 in every thousand (2.0%) of the population.

## What sort of people get CFS/ME?

CFS/ME can occur at any age and can affect people with all sorts of occupations or income levels. Specialized hospital clinics do tend to have a higher proportion of well-educated, professional patients, but that may be due to those people's greater ability to get themselves referred to such clinics.

CFS/ME does seem to occur more often in women than in men, though it is not clear why this should be so.

## What is the outcome (or 'prognosis') of CFS/ME?

The majority of people with CFS/ME improve. The illness is usually at its worst in the first few months and tends to improve thereafter. It is important to stress that for most people this illness does not lead to long-term severe disability. However, recovery can be a slow process and often takes the form of a frustrating 'up and down' pattern of improvements and setbacks.

Some people make a complete recovery, while others feel improved but would not regard themselves as having returned to full health. Unfortunately, a minority of people do remain chronically ill for reasons that are not well understood. These differing outcomes may reflect different types of CFS/ME. They probably also reflect the different ways in which patients respond to and cope with the illness. By managing your illness as well as possible, you will give yourself the best chance of improvement and recovery. We discuss what 'good management' means in the second section of this book.

---

Fatigue is very common in the general population. Severe, chronic, disabling fatigue is much less common. It can be a symptom of a number of illnesses, especially stress and depression. People who are suffering from severe fatigue may get a diagnosis of CFS/ME if they have:

◆ severe fatigue that limits their ability to do things

◆ a number of other symptoms

◆ no other known medical condition that could produce similar symptoms.

CFS/ME can affect anyone, although it is more common in women. Most people improve, although the degree of recovery varies. You can give yourself the best chance of improvement by following the advice included in Section 2 of this book.

---

# 4

# How is a diagnosis of CFS/ME made?

 Key points

- A diagnosis of CFS/ME is made when:

    - the typical symptoms are present

    - other diseases that could cause severe, chronic fatigue are excluded

- This is done by taking a history, doing a physical examination, and by ordering some laboratory tests

- If the test results are 'normal' this does **not** mean that you are not ill, just that you don't have the disease that the test detects

A diagnosis of CFS/ME is made on the basis of what the patient says—that is on their symptoms and the history of their illness. There are no findings on examination (clinical signs) in CFS/ME and so far there is no medical test. A full history, physical examination, and laboratory investigations or 'tests' are important, however, to exclude other conditions that could be causing the symptoms.

## Ruling out other conditions

To do this, the doctor assessing you will listen to your history, examine you, and arrange any necessary tests. In this way he or she will rule out other diseases. This is important. If you were found to have another disease that is readily treatable or even life threatening (which CFS/ME is not), you would receive different treatment. The list of conditions that can cause symptoms similar to those of CFS/ME is a long one. However, your doctor will be unlikely to need to ask questions about or do tests for **all** of these conditions. This would be time consuming, potentially hazardous to you, and very expensive. Instead, he or she will only test for those conditions which are either very common or which your history (and physical examination) suggest as a possible explanation for the symptoms in your case. The most important way of finding out what is wrong is by asking the patient about their illness—what is called 'taking a history'.

## Further history

The doctor may want to ask you about other symptoms in order to obtain more information to help make a diagnosis. As depression and anxiety are among the most common causes of fatigue, your doctor is also likely to consider whether these could be a factor in your case and to ask about other symptoms that could suggest these (see Chapters 5 and 22). Having depression or anxiety does not mean that you cannot also have CFS—but it makes sense to diagnose and treat these conditions if present and then see what symptoms are left. Your doctor will also ask about other symptoms that might suggest other diseases.

## Physical examination

Having taken a history, the doctor will usually conduct a physical examination. Depending on what he or she has learned from the history this may be a very limited one or may be a full examination requiring that you undress.

## Laboratory tests

Some very common illnesses should probably be tested for in everyone who has chronic fatigue. These are anaemia, evidence of inflammation or infection, disturbance of blood chemistry due to liver, kidney, or hormonal dysfunction, a low level of thyroid hormone, and diabetes mellitus. The tests for these are:

| Test | What it rules out |
|---|---|
| Full blood count | Anaemia |
| | Infection |
| ESR (erythrocyte sedimentation rate) | Infection or inflammation |
| CRP (C-reactive protein) | |

*(continued)*

| Test | What it rules out |
|---|---|
| Urea and electrolytes | Kidney problems. Problems with the level of sodium and potassium in the blood |
| Liver function tests | Problems with the liver |
| T3/T4/TSH | Problems with the thyroid gland |
| Urine/blood glucose | Diabetes mellitus |

T3, triiodothyronine; T4, thyroxine; TSH, thyroid-stimulating hormone.

## Other conditions that can cause fatigue

There are other less common conditions that may need to be excluded in a few people. The list is long. In fact, most known diseases can cause fatigue. However, these less common diseases are only rarely found in people with the typical symptoms of CFS/ME, and most of these diseases are treatable. We cannot provide a complete list but have given some examples of medical conditions that cause fatigue and might be considered by your doctor:

- If you have a lot of joint and muscle pain, your doctor may do tests for a range of rheumatic diseases. Rarer 'autoimmune' diseases (where the body's own immune system causes damage to bodily organs) often cause joint pain and fatigue. Your doctors will usually be alerted to this possibility by findings on examination or from standard blood tests.

- Some gastrointestinal diseases may lead to fatigue. They usually cause diarrhoea and weight loss. If you have predominant gastric symptoms, your doctor may arrange for tests to exclude such conditions. One such condition is coeliac disease, which is caused by inflammation of the small intestine due to a reaction to the gluten in certain cereals (wheat, barley, and rye). The treatment is a gluten-free diet and is usually completely effective.

- Neurological diseases can present with fatigue. Multiple sclerosis usually causes loss of power or sensation in part of the body and can also cause fatigue. Myasthenia gravis is a rare condition in which there is a problem between muscles and the nerves that make them work. It causes weakness. Both have treatments.

- Hormonal conditions can lead to fatigue. A routine test of urine or blood glucose for diabetes may be appropriate, as may a blood test for an underactive thyroid gland. An endocrine condition called Addison's disease (due to inadequate functioning of the adrenal gland) also causes fatigue, but is very rare. Giving the missing hormone can treat all these conditions.

♦ Infections can certainly cause fatigue. Examples include viral hepatitis, Lyme disease, glandular fever (Epstein–Barr virus), and Q fever. These infections can trigger fatigue. Less commonly they can persist. They are relatively uncommon causes of chronic fatigue.

♦ Severe sleep problems, such as a condition called sleep apnoea syndrome, can cause daytime fatigue, mainly sleepiness. Sleep apnoea is when a person stops breathing briefly many times during the night, often in association with loud snoring. It is diagnosed by having sleep and breathing measured overnight in a sleep laboratory. It can be treated.

### Expensive and sophisticated tests

If your doctor suspects that you might be suffering from another condition, further specialist tests might be done. For example, if there is something that suggests you could have a problem with the nerves in your arms or legs, electrical equipment may be used to test the nerves (this is called neurophysiological testing). If a disease is suspected which would have a visible effect on the brain, a CT (computed tomography) or an MRI (magnetic resonance imaging) scan might be done to obtain a picture of the brain. These scans are **not** a test for CFS/ME, as the results in patients with the illness are typically normal. They do, however, provide a means of excluding other brain diseases. MRI scans are particularly sensitive at detecting multiple sclerosis (MS).

# A reassuring note

Research shows that once patients who have the symptoms of CFS/ME have been seen and assessed by a doctor, the chance that other possible causes have been missed is small. Once patients have been seen by several doctors, that chance becomes even smaller. However, it is not possible to exclude all diseases conclusively. So, if your symptoms change, it may be wise to tell your doctor and not to assume automatically that every new symptom is due to CFS/ME. On the other hand, it really is unhelpful to focus too much on your symptoms. This simply holds you back from recovery and gets in the way of enjoying life.

# After the tests

When your doctor has ruled out all the other things that might be causing the symptoms he or she can say that it is probably CFS. If you had a viral infection at the beginning of your illness, your doctor may call it post-viral fatigue syndrome (PVFS).

You may find it helpful to ask your doctor what tests have been performed and what has been ruled out. At least then you will know what you do **not** have. Do remember that if your doctor says, 'all the tests are normal' he or she is **not** saying that you are not feeling ill. It just means that you do not have any of the medical conditions that these tests reveal. The lack of a definitive medical test for CFS/ME does not mean that the illness does not exist, or that it is 'all in your mind'.

Some doctors are reluctant to give patients a diagnosis of CFS because they believe that not enough is known about it and that it is not a proper or helpful diagnosis. This is understandable from the doctor's point of view, but it often leaves patients in a difficult position. It is hard for anyone to make sense of their illness or to deal with it in the best way without a diagnosis. If your doctor prefers not to make a diagnosis, it may be helpful to explain this to him or her.

A diagnosis of CFS/ME is made by excluding other diseases that might cause severe chronic fatigue and associated symptoms. Most common conditions causing similar symptoms can be ruled out by asking you questions, examining you, and conducting simple blood or urine tests. Your doctor may test for other rarer conditions if there is something in your history, symptoms, or examination that suggests this as a possibility. Although there is no definitive medical test for CFS/ME, this does not mean that it is 'all in your mind'. All illnesses, including CFS/ME, have physical, psychological, and social aspects.

# 5

# What other conditions is CFS/ME linked to?

> ### ➡ Key points
>
> ◆ People with the symptoms of CFS/ME may be given other diagnoses
>
> ◆ These other diagnoses may be different labels for the same illness
>
> ◆ Whatever the diagnosis, these symptoms tend to respond to the self-help approach outlined in Section 2

People who are diagnosed as having CFS/ME may have other symptoms. A doctor may make other diagnoses (offer other 'labels') for these symptoms. These diagnoses may include one or more of the following:

◆ fibromyalgia (FMS)

◆ irritable bowel syndrome (IBS)

◆ pre-menstrual syndrome (PMS)

◆ non-cardiac chest pain

◆ anxiety and panic

◆ depression

◆ other more controversial diagnoses.

# Fibromyalgia (FMS)

Where aches and pains are prominent without evidence of muscle or joint disease, a diagnosis of fibromyalgia (previously called fibrositis) may be made, especially if there are 'tender spots' in certain places on the body. FMS is so closely related to CFS that it has been suggested that CFS/ME and FMS are in fact the same condition. They certainly overlap, and many people with CFS/ME also meet the diagnostic criteria for FMS, and vice versa. CFS/ME is the diagnosis given when the person complains more of fatigue than pain and FMS when the problem is more pain than fatigue. Most people with CFS/ME and FMS have both fatigue and pain.

Furthermore, similar treatments have been found to help both conditions—pacing activities, graded increases in physical activity, and cognitive–behavioural therapy, as well as the so-called 'antidepressant' drugs such as amitriptyline (Tryptizol or Elavil). The main difference is that the people with FMS may benefit more from painkilling medicines.

# Irritable bowel syndrome (IBS)

Problems with digestion and bowel functioning are common in the general population. They seem to be particularly common in people with a diagnosis of CFS/ME. Your doctor should be able to rule out treatable conditions such as coeliac disease (see Chapter 4) and other inflammations of the bowel.

The symptoms typical of IBS are altered bowel habit, bloating, and 'colicky' abdominal pains. Like CFS the diagnosis is made principally by exclusion of other medical causes of the symptoms. The cause is unknown. Dietary changes (such as adding roughage to the diet) sometimes help. The symptoms may, at least in part, be stress related. Learning to relax, to manage stress, and to reduce worry often helps.

# Pre-menstrual syndrome/tension (PMS/PMT)

Some women report a worsening of fatigue and other symptoms of CFS/ME and increased irritability in the days leading up to their menstrual period. They may be given a diagnosis of PMS/PMT. A variety of treatments have been suggested for this syndrome. There is evidence that the so-called 'antidepressant' drugs, especially SSRIs (selective serotonin reuptake inhibitors) such as fluoxetine (Prozac) are effective for many with this syndrome. Exercise has also been shown to help. Recognizing that these are the the most difficult days of the month can be useful to you so that you can pace yourself through them carefully. However, we suggest that you do not just focus on these days but apply the more general approaches we describe *every day*.

# Non-cardiac or 'atypical' chest pain and palpitations

Pains in the chest or an awareness of the heart beating are common symptoms. Because they suggest a problem with the heart, these symptoms can be particularly frightening. If you suffer from these symptoms, it is wise to see a doctor to ensure that they are not due to heart disease. Heart disease is common in our society and therefore needs to be excluded. Your doctor may wish to arrange tests such as an electrocardiogram and sometimes an exercise test. In most cases, however, particularly in younger people, the heart will be found to be healthy.

'Stress', anxiety, and panic can cause these symptoms, and they are often associated with panic (see below). Once a person has experienced chest pain, it can be made worse by worry about the symptoms themselves. Even after heart disease has been excluded, some people may require specific psychological help to manage these symptoms. The approach described in this book should also be helpful.

# Anxiety and panic attacks

Worry, stress, anxiety, and panic attacks can all cause **physical** symptoms. They do this by activating the body's 'alarm system'—preparing it to fight or run away. This system includes the sympathetic part of the nervous system and the release of a hormone called adrenaline (epinephrine). Activation of it, such as occurs in anxiety and panic, causes a person to breathe more quickly, to have a faster heartbeat, and to tense their muscles. Repeated activation of this alarm system can produce profound fatigue.

The physical symptoms of anxiety and panic can be frightening in themselves, especially if they lead the person to fear that they have a life-threatening disease (e.g. chest pains suggesting a problem with the heart as described above). This fear of disease can cause a vicious circle which works like this: anxiety produces physical symptoms, the sufferer worries that these physical symptoms mean they have serious disease, and gets more anxious, which leads to them having even more symptoms. People who have severe anxiety and panic may require help from a doctor or psychologist (for drug treatment and/or specialist psychological treatment).

# Depressive illness

It may surprise you to hear that depression is commonly associated with **physical** symptoms, not just emotional ones. These can include fatigue, muscle pain, and sleep problems. If symptoms of depression are present as well as those suggesting CFS/ME, it does not necessarily mean that the illness is 'really' just depression—but it does strongly suggest that treatment of depression will help and may reduce physical symptoms as well as emotional ones. Whatever else is wrong, it is better not to be depressed. Depression usually gets better if treated with antidepressant drugs or with cognitive–behavioural therapy. The self-help approaches described in Chapter 22 are also likely to be useful for depression.

# Controversial diagnoses

There are other diagnoses given to people with symptoms of CFS/ME with names that not only describe the symptoms, but also imply a specific cause. This makes them controversial if the suggested cause is not generally agreed. These controversial syndromes include multiple chemical sensitivity (MCS), candidiasis (widespread infection with a yeast called *Candida albicans*), hypoglycaemia (low blood sugar), and chronic Lyme disease. Whilst there is no doubt that chemicals, *Candida albicans* infection, hypoglycaemia, and Lyme disease can cause symptoms, research suggests that it is very unlikely that they are causing the symptoms in most patients with symptoms of CFS/ME.

We therefore urge you to be very cautious about accepting these diagnoses or taking treatment based on them.

## Multiple chemical sensitivity (MCS)

Those who believe in multiple chemical sensitivity as a cause of symptoms suggest that if symptoms appear to be associated with exposure to one or more chemicals, such chemicals are the cause. Whilst the reality of the symptoms is not in doubt, the suggestion that the chemical causes them is unproven. Those who make this diagnosis commonly advocate avoidance of all situations that have been associated with symptoms. This treatment may help reduce symptoms in the short term because it reduces anxiety about exposing oneself to chemicals. However, it also has a major impact on social contact and quality of life. It may also make symptoms worse in the longer term. It should not be undertaken lightly and we do not recommend it.

## Systemic candidiasis (yeast infection)

*Candida albicans* is a yeast, which can be a cause of vaginal discharge (thrush) and white sore patches in the mouth and skin. All of these can be treated by the use of antifungal drugs such as clotrimazole (Canesten or Lotrimin) or nystatin (Nystan or Nilstat).

However, the suggestion that an 'overgrowth' of *Candida* in the bowel or blood is a common cause of the symptoms of CFS/ME is not supported by evidence. The recommended treatment usually involves drastic changes in diet, the use of supplements and probiotics, and sometimes also antifungal drugs such as nystatin. The dietary changes can be difficult and interfere with adequate nutrition. The supplements recommended can be very expensive. Antifungal drugs can be toxic. We cannot recommend this form of treatment.

## Food allergy and sensitivity

Some people blame illness on what they eat and some aspects of diet can lead to diseases. Many people with CFS/ME feel that certain foods worsen their symptoms for reasons that are not well understood. Food allergies exist. Some people do have true allergies to foods such as peanuts, and get severe reactions if they are exposed to them. If you do get definite symptoms of allergy—such as tingling and swelling of the tongue and lips, wheezing, or rash—this is potentially life threatening and you should see your doctor.

However, food allergy is almost certainly not a major cause of the symptoms of CFS/ME. Whatever some therapists may say, there is no good evidence that CFS/ME is due to food sensitivity. If you feel better avoiding certain foods it may be reasonable to exclude them from your diet. But do be careful—excluding too many foods may put your nutrition at risk and can certainly reduce your quality of life.

## Hypoglycaemia (low blood sugar)

Low blood sugar is a potential problem for people being treated for diabetes mellitus where the treatment may reduce the blood sugar more than necessary.

However, there is very little evidence that other people have symptoms caused by low blood sugar. There is no good evidence that low blood sugar is a cause of CFS/ME. Excessive sugar intake with the idea of combating 'low blood sugar' is not justified and may cause weight gain.

## Chronic Lyme disease

Lyme disease is an illness caused by infection with a bacterium (*Borrelia burgdorferi*) that is caught by being bitten by a tick. It causes an acute severe illness with a skin rash, and usually obvious abnormalities on tests; it is treated by antibiotics. It has been suggested that some people with the fatigue and muscle aches typical of CFS/ME really have chronic untreated Lyme disease.

However, whilst Lyme disease clearly exists, and is a serious illness, it is now thought very unlikely that chronic Lyme disease is a cause of CFS/ME. Furthermore, the often prolonged courses of high-dose antibiotics are almost certainly unjustified and are likely to have adverse effects. If you have been in a part of the world, such as certain parts of the USA, where Lyme disease is common and you become ill, it is important to seek medical attention. However, if you have symptoms of CFS/ME it is very unlikely that these are due to the infection that causes Lyme disease. We have included a paper about Lyme disease in Appendix 3.

# What do I do if I have been given one of these diagnoses?

Discuss it with your doctor. If you also have CFS/ME, the main thing to recognize is that being given one of these diagnoses does not necessarily mean that you have more than one problem—rather it is likely that each group of symptoms represents different aspects of a common problem. Which label you are given may depend to some degree on which specialist you see—a rheumatologist might use the label fibromyalgia, whilst a gastroenterologist might use the label irritable bowel syndrome. Furthermore, although there are specific treatments recommended for some of these conditions, they are all likely to be helped by the self-help approach we outline in this book.

> If you have fatigue and other symptoms you may have been given a diagnosis of CFS/ME. You may also be told that you have another diagnosis. If this is of one of the conditions we have talked about in this chapter, it is probably another name for the same problem rather than something new. The suggestions we make in this book are likely to be useful for managing any of these conditions, so do not let labels confuse you or prevent you from working to manage your symptoms. Some of the better understood conditions such as depression, anxiety, and panic respond to specific medical and psychological treatment. If you think you have one of these, you should discuss it with your doctor.

# 6

# What do we know about CFS/ME?

> ### ⊙ Key points
>
> ◆ Much research into CFS/ME has been done to answer questions such as who gets it, what is the cause, and whether there is a test. However, so far there have been few clear answers
>
> ◆ When reading the published research, you should be sceptical and try to judge the soundness of the evidence yourself
>
> ◆ Current research is focusing mainly on how changes in the way the brain works may cause the symptoms of CFS/ME

There has already been a great deal of research into CFS/ME. The aims have been to find out how many people have CFS/ME and the factors associated with it (epidemiology), to understand the causes (aetiology), and to find a test which will positively diagnose the condition (diagnostic test). Research is of course ultimately devoted to finding an effective treatment. Research into treatment (clinical trials) is discussed in Chapter 8.

Before we go on to discuss what research has been done and is being done, as well as likely directions for future research, we need to give you a warning. You do need to be sceptical when reading about 'new research into CFS/ME', particularly research that is heralded as 'finding the cause of the illness', 'finding a diagnostic marker for the illness', or 'finding a cure'. The process of doing scientific research is a slow and difficult one. Progress in science is largely about trial and error—many findings are later disproved and it can be hard to know which findings will stand the test of time. A great deal of research is published. It has been said that we could reduce the confusion by discarding half the published research—the problem is we do not know which half!

So, before having your hopes falsely raised, please read the following. It may also be useful to combat over-enthusiasm for new findings and treatment amongst family and friends:

♦ Before any meaningful research can be done, it is important that different researchers work out how to make sure they are studying the same illness. Hence the importance of a definition of CFS with clear guidance on how to decide whether a patient meets the definition (see Chapter 3). Published research must be clear about exactly what illness the findings refer to.

♦ Beware of any research findings that appear in the media or popular magazines before they have been published in a reputable scientific journal. Before doctors and scientists can get research findings published in such journals they have to have their work reviewed by other scientists (this is called peer review) as well as by the editor of the journal. This is a basic safeguard against faulty or misleading findings being published. However, it is not infallible. Even if something gets published in a scientific journal, it does not necessarily mean that it is true. And of course, some journals have more rigorous procedures and are more reputable than others!

♦ Even with this basic safeguard of peer review, any finding that cannot be repeated by other scientists is unlikely to be worth much. The field of CFS/ME is sadly littered with published observations (often heralded as 'breakthroughs') that have subsequently not been confirmed by other researchers.

♦ 'Association' does not necessarily mean 'cause'. Just because a chemical or some other measure is increased or decreased in people with CFS/ME does not mean that this is the 'cause' of CFS/ME. There can be other explanations. In one famous study of another illness, a change in the urine that was thought to represent the chemical cause of that illness turned out to be an effect of the hospital diet!

♦ Scientific findings are often not clinically relevant. Even if they are true, many, if not most, research findings do not have any immediate relevance to the investigation and treatment of individual patients.

♦ Science is not just a laboratory exercise. Science is a method of finding the truth by carefully collecting and weighing evidence (as opposed to guess work, prejudice, or dogma). This discipline of thought is just as important in the clinical evaluation of patients and treatment as it is to the study of cells in a laboratory.

Having outlined some of the limitations and hazards of research, we can tell you something about what has been found so far. We have also included books and published papers in our reading list that can give you more details of research into CFS/ME (Appendix 3).

# Research into CFS/ME in populations (epidemiology)

Epidemiology can tell us how many people in the population have a disease (how many cases), what factors are associated with it, and what the outcome is for people suffering from that disease. There has been a limited amount of epidemiological research into CFS/ME. Just how common it is found to be (its prevalence) depends on exactly how a 'case' of CFS/ME is defined. The rates reported therefore vary. Reported figures are between 0.2 and 2% of the population. These studies show that CFS/ME occurs in all social classes but is more common in women—the reason for this is unknown. The peak age of onset is about 30 years, but all ages can be affected. Outcome studies suggest that most patients do improve rather than deteriorate, and that by 5 years after onset half feel they have recovered.

# Research into the cause of CFS/ME (aetiology)

This section describes what has been found out about possible causes of CFS/ME. When we talk about 'cause', we mean both what might have started off the illness and what might be keeping it going (read more about this in the section on the 'three Ps' in Chapter 7).

There have been many studies into the causes of CFS/ME. These are summarized briefly under a number of headings:

## Genes

As our body is built from a blueprint inherited from our parents and coded in our genes, it is to be expected that vulnerability to various illnesses will be inherited from our parents. It is unlikely that CFS/ME would be an exception. Genetic studies of large numbers of patients have indeed found that some people have a modestly greater inherited vulnerability to CFS/ME than others. However, despite much interest in the area, no specific genes have so far been reliably found to be associated with CFS/ME and there is no genetic test.

## Infection and the immune system

There has been a great deal of research in this area. Because many people with CFS/ME say that it started with a 'virus' infection, this has seemed an obvious place to begin. One question is whether people who get any sort of infection are more likely to get CFS/ME; perhaps surprisingly they do not seem to be. Another question is whether people who are infected with certain specific infections are more likely to get CFS/ME. The infectious agents studied include the Epstein–Barr virus (that causes glandular fever) and the Q fever agent. There is evidence that people who get these infections are more likely to go on to get CFS/ME, but how the infection does this remains uncertain. Whilst some virus infections may **trigger** CFS/ME in certain people, the symptoms of CFS/ME do not seem to be caused by a persistent virus infection. Treating people with CFS/ME using the few drugs available that kill viruses does not work.

It has also been suggested that an alteration in the body's immune system could be responsible for the symptoms of CFS/ME. A good deal of work has been carried out to look for evidence of this. The immune system seems to be slightly abnormal in some patients (but not all). However, the importance of these findings is still unclear. The changes found are relatively small and can occur in other illnesses such as depression. It is not clear that they cause the symptoms of CFS/ME. However, there are links between the immune system and the brain (see below) that may yet turn out to be important. Research continues in this field.

## Muscles

As so many people with CFS/ME report muscle pain and muscle weakness, researchers have looked to see if they can find a problem with the muscles. However, the muscles seem to be normal. Rather it is more likely that the problem is in the nervous system and how messages to and from the muscles are sent and received by the brain (see below).

## The brain

The common symptoms of CFS/ME are fatigue, sleep disturbance, and poor concentration. There is also some evidence that people with CFS/ME find it more difficult to do complex mental tasks. These symptoms point to a problem with the brain. The structure of the brains of people with CFS/ME has been studied using 'scans' CT (computerized tomography), MRI (magnetic resonance imaging), and PET (positron emission tomography). Most doctors believe that the structure of the brain is normal in patients with CFS/ME—that is there is no evidence of brain damage. If there are no problems in the structure of the brain the problem is in how it is working—its functioning. There is some evidence for this. Some scans (SPECT [single photon emission computed tomography] and PET) look at the functioning of the brain by measuring how much blood each bit of the brain is using, which reflects how hard it is working. Some of the studies that used these scans have reported a slightly lower blood flow (hypoperfusion) in certain areas of the brain (though different researchers have found this in different areas), suggesting that there may be changes in brain functioning in patients with CFS/ME. They do not, as some have suggested, indicate that blood vessels are blocked in CFS/ME.

Another way to find out about brain functioning is to do tests that tell us about the levels of different neurotransmitters (the chemicals that enable brain cells to talk to each other). Some studies have found these to be abnormal in some patients with CFS/ME. In particular, one area of the brain where these neurotransmitters may be abnormal is the hypothalamus. This is a small but particularly important part of the brain that controls hormones via the pituitary gland. There is some evidence that suggests that this system is not functioning quite normally in people with CFS/ME (see stress hormones below). There is also evidence that these changes may differ from those usually seen in people who are depressed (see below).

## Stress

Stress is the name given to physical, psychological, and social pressures on a person that make them feel 'stressed' or under strain. Stressors can range from simple environmental factors such as noise, to excessive worry about things, to being badly treated by other people. Illness itself can be stressful. The symptoms of being under stress include fatigue, sleep disturbance, irritability, depression, and anxiety. Stress has major effects on the body. In particular it has effects on the nervous and hormonal systems, especially on the release of cortisol from the adrenal gland (see below). Patients with CFS/ME commonly report suffering a period of stress prior to the onset of the illness. Does stress cause CFS? Stress can be the trigger for a wide range of illnesses and it is still unclear why some people get CFS/ME after stress whilst others do not. Stress may only be a cause in people who also have some other factor such as an infection. In summary, whilst most clinicians think stress is an important factor in many people, the scientific evidence for this is limited. More research is needed.

## Stress hormones

When we are stressed—physically or mentally—our brain tells our adrenal glands to increase the level of cortisol in our blood. This is done by a part of the brain called the hypothalamus, which changes the chemicals released into the blood by the pituitary gland. This gland in turn controls the adrenal gland output of cortisol. The whole system is called the hypothalamic–pituitary–adrenal (HPA) axis. People who have a faulty HPA axis (such as those with Addison's disease) often feel severely fatigued. It has therefore been suggested that it may be the brain's control of stress hormones that is defective in CFS/ME. There is some evidence for this, but the abnormalities found so far are small. A group of people with CFS/ME may have *on average* a lower level of stress hormones than healthy people; however, this does not mean that this difference will be detectable in all *individuals*. Furthermore, the benefits of giving cortisol as a medicine to people with CFS/ME remain unclear, and can be harmful. We do not therefore recommend steroids as a treatment for CFS/ME.

## Problems with the body clock—circadian rhythm and sleep

People with CFS/ME commonly report disturbed sleep, most commonly broken and unrefreshing sleep and altered times of sleep. It seems obvious to suggest that poor sleep may lead to increased fatigue. There has been some research into the sleep problems experienced by many people with CFS/ME and whether these are the cause of fatigue. The results seem to indicate that whilst disturbed sleep and abnormal sleep/wake rhythms may contribute to fatigue, muscle pain, and poor concentration, they are not the basic cause of the illness. However, research continues.

## Changes in blood pressure—postural hypotension

When we stand up, our blood pressure tends to drop briefly. It has been found that a proportion of patients with CFS/ME show an unusually large drop in their blood pressure when moving from lying to standing. This has been investigated by laying them on a special table that tilts (a tilt table). Blood pressure and symptoms are monitored whilst the tilt table is moved from horizontal to vertical. There is a suggestion from these experiments that dizziness and fatigue are made worse in some patients when they are standing up (and their blood pressure goes down). This finding is of interest and could be due to changes in brain function. However, it is still unclear just how common this problem really is in people with CFS/ME and whether it is a cause of the illness, or simply an effect of being ill and less active.

## The effects of inactivity

We all need rest, but research has shown that too much rest can be harmful. Prolonged inactivity, even in fit persons, can itself cause fatigue and make it harder to be active. It can also have very profound effects on the body and mind, such as changes in blood-pressure regulation leading to postural hypotension (as above), changes in the body's ability to tolerate activity, changed temperature regulation, and actual physical changes in the functioning and bulk of muscles. Some people with CFS/ME become persistently inactive, and for them it is likely that inactivity contributes to their symptoms. Many others appear to become trapped in an oscillation between inactivity and activity. The effects of this oscillating pattern of activity and inactivity are poorly understood. It would appear, however, not to help the body regain its capacity for normal activity.

## Depression and anxiety

Many studies have found that depression and anxiety are very common in people with CFS/ME. It has even been suggested that depression is the cause of CFS/ME. It is true that it can be very hard to sort out whether symptoms such as fatigue, muscle pain, and poor concentration are due to depression and/or anxiety or to CFS/ME. However, this is not the same as asking whether depression actually causes CFS/ME. In fact that is probably not even a sensible question. This is because both depression and CSF/ME are diagnosed purely on the basis of the symptoms a person has—to say that depression causes CFS is like saying that symptoms cause symptoms!

Another way to look at this question is to ask whether the *causes* of CFS/ME are the same as the causes of depression. To some extent they probably are, as stress and the resulting changes in the functioning of the brain and hormone levels seem to play a role in both. In other ways they are probably not, as the actual changes observed in brain and hormonal function are different—for example the stress hormone cortisol tends to be increased in people with depression but decreased in people with CFS/ME.

It is also reasonable to expect that the experience of CFS/ME could cause depression. If you have an illness over which you believe you have no personal control, it is likely to make you feel helpless and hopeless about the outcome. A feeling of helplessness and hopelessness is in turn one of the recognized causes of depression.

Whilst depression/anxiety can be very hard to disentangle, in practice the problem is easier. Depression can be treated, so if there is any doubt it is often wise to try a treatment for depression and see if it helps.

## Ways of understanding and coping with CFS/ME

There is evidence that people who believe very strongly that their illness is a disease caused by factors outside their control, and who deny the importance of psychological or social factors in their illness, have a worse outcome. A belief that the symptoms caused by activity are dangerous also seems to be associated with greater disability. These research findings could mean that these people simply have a more severe physical illness. However, that does not seem to be the reason. Rather it seems more likely that this way of thinking about the illness leads people to cope in ways that do not encourage recovery—for example by resting, avoiding any activity that seems to make symptoms worse, not getting treatment for depression, or not working on their rehabilitation.

## The behaviour of other people

People are not simply individuals. They relate to and are influenced by the people about them—family, friends, doctors, officials, and those around them at work. These social factors can have an influence on how ill a person with CFS/ME feels and what they are able to achieve. There is less research into this aspect of CFS/ME, but most patients and doctors are aware of its importance. There is research into patients' experiences of CFS/ME that has illustrated just how difficult it is to manage any illness well in a climate of disbelief, particularly if that disbelief is coming from those close to you. If those around you do not accept or understand your illness, it can be much more difficult to cope effectively. You may find yourself with a need to demonstrate repeatedly to others just how bad you are feeling. Self-doubt may also creep in, fuelling premature attempts to 'behave normally'. (We talk about ways to explain an 'invisible illness' in Chapter 25.)

At the other extreme, excessive protectiveness by those close to you can be a real problem. Studies of patients with chronic pain have shown how well-meaning help from others can make a person more disabled than they need to be. Clinical studies suggest that, in some cases, a partner or parent may have found a role for him or herself in being a carer and so apply subtle and perhaps unconscious pressures on the sufferer to be dependent on them.

Finally, if a person has had to give up employment and exist on benefits or insurance payments, it can be difficult to make the switch back to working. Studies of other chronic illnesses, such as back pain, show that when people are off work for a long time it becomes unlikely that they will return. That is probably because managing the transition from illness to working—especially if you would have to function at your previous level—can be very difficult.

# Research into a 'test' for CFS/ME (diagnostic test)

A diagnostic test has great appeal. It would counter the 'all in the mind' accusation. It might make diagnosis easier and more reliable. But unless it leads to a treatment, its value is limited. None of the findings listed above are sufficiently specific to this illness to function as a 'test'. Indeed if, as is suspected, CFS/ME is in fact caused by a variety of physical factors, it is likely that only a subgroup of patients would be positive on any one single test. This would raise issues for those who were test-negative. At present there is no established test or 'marker' for CFS/ME.

## Future directions

Where do we go from here? Probably much of the research being done will continue to explore many of the ideas described above using increasingly sophisticated techniques. There is likely to be more research attempting to differentiate between subgroups of the illness—what are the different types and should there be different treatments for different subgroups? Another potentially useful direction for research is to study those factors that are common to all chronic illnesses, such as the effects of reduced activity.

What is clear is that the future focus of research is likely to be on the brain and nervous system. On the one hand, the brain affects the function of the endocrine and immune systems. On the other hand, the state and functioning of the brain are of course affected by what a person thinks and does and by the behaviour of others. A focus on the brain in research might be what unifies the study of the mind and the body in CFS/ME.

> Much research into CFS/ME has already been done. So far this research has produced as many questions as answers. It is important that CFS/ME sufferers should be sceptical about some of the published research and try to judge the soundness of the evidence. Current research is focusing on the brain, on how reversible changes in the brain cause illness, and how social and psychological factors affect the brain.

# 7

# Making sense of what we know about the causes of CFS/ME: who gets it, what triggers it, and why don't people get better?

## ➔ Key points

◆ It is unlikely that there is one single cause of CFS/ME

◆ It may be more useful to look at many causes grouped as the 'three Ps'

    ◆ Predisposing—what makes a person more likely to get CFS/ME

    ◆ Precipitating—what might have triggered the illness

    ◆ Perpetuating—what might be keeping the illness going

We want facts, but unfortunately this chapter is going to be full of 'maybes'. In spite of all the research that has been done, there are few definite facts. No one single cause for CFS/ME has been identified. In fact, most experts think that there are probably several routes into the illness and that yet other factors keeping it going once it has begun. Over the years, many researchers have enthusiastically pursued theories that they have hoped would be 'the cause'. To date, none of these has achieved general acceptance. Most researchers now believe that CFS/ME will ultimately be found to include a number of separate conditions. This means that not all people who have had a diagnosis of CFS/ME may have the same illness.

# A way of thinking about cause—the 'three Ps'

It has been suggested that looking for a single cause, even in one individual, may be a mistake. Instead, it may be more helpful to look for a number of causes. These causes may also play different roles. These roles can usefully be grouped into three categories, which are sometimes called the 'three Ps'. These refer to what makes a person more likely to get CFS/ME (Predisposing), what triggers the illness (Precipitating), and what keeps it going once established— the obstacles to recovery (Perpetuating). This way of looking at the illness may be less instantly appealing than the idea of a single cause. However, it does have the advantage of opening up a much wider way of thinking about cause, which in turn offers more ways that an individual can be helped or can help himself or herself.

## Predisposing factors: who gets it?

Relatively little is known about the factors that make a person more likely to develop CFS/ME. Doctors working in specialized clinics may recognize that some things frequently occur in their patients' medical histories, but these factors do not occur in everyone. An overactive or striving lifestyle with inadequate time for rest and reflection leading to chronic stress has been suggested as one predisposing factor. Stress over a long period may also predispose some people to CFS/ME. A previous history of depression also predisposes to CFS/ME. There is some evidence for genetic factors as well. However, none of these factors is enough in itself to explain why one person develops CFS/ME whilst another apparently similar person does not.

## Precipitating factors: what triggers it?

Why might people who are predisposed to getting CFS/ME go on to develop the illness? Many, but not all, people with CFS/ME report that their illness had a sudden onset, often following an acute viral-type illness. A virus infection may act as a trigger for the illness in some people. Severe emotional upset such as bereavement, or an accident or operation, or some kind of trauma may be a trigger in others. It is possible that it is a combination of these factors that is important. In some people, the illness just gradually develops with no apparent trigger.

### Perpetuating factors: what keeps it going?

It is natural for anyone to feel a need to understand why they **became** ill, but in practical terms it is more important to identify things that are **keeping** them ill and preventing a natural improvement or recovery. This is because they are the targets for treatments. The perpetuating factors may be different from the precipitating factors. For example, a virus infection may have precipitated the illness, but by a year later the virus has long gone and other factors are preventing recovery.

The factors perpetuating CFS are only partially understood, and various theories have been suggested. None has so far been proved to be definitely true. However, in all chronic illness, in general, there is evidence that a number of factors can perpetuate symptoms and disability. In CFS/ME these might include biological changes such as changes in the functioning of the brain and HPA (hypothalamic–pituitary–adrenal) axis, psychological factors such as unhelpful thinking about symptoms, and social factors such as other people's lack of understanding of the illness.

# A multifactorial theory of the perpetuation of CFS/ME

We do not know for certain what perpetuates CFS/ME. However,a combination of evidence from research into CFS/ME and from research into related conditions such as chronic pain supports the following ideas. Manydoctors and therapists (though not all) accept these ideas, which haveled to the development of useful treatments for CFS/ME such as cognitive–behavioural therapy and graded exercise therapy. These are currently the most effective treatments for CFS/ME. This multifactorial theory suggests that:

1. Many different factors (physical, psychological, and social) can perpetuate CFS.

2. Different combinations of factors may be important in different people.

3. These factors may interact to form vicious circles, trapping the person in disability.

4. Removing or reducing these perpetuating factors by breaking the vicious circles can aid recovery.

## Factors that may perpetuate CFS/ME

The factors that can probably perpetuate CFS/ME include the biological, psychological, and social aspects of the illness listed below:

## Biological

- Abnormal brain functioning

- Altered stress hormones

- Sleep disturbance

- Effect of inactivity

- Possibly other changes such as immune activation.

## Psychological

- Unhelpful beliefs about the illness such as 'There is nothing I can do'

- Unhelpful coping behaviours such as excessive rest, avoidance of activity, or an oscillating level of activity

- Negative mood such as depression and anxiety

- More general factors such as a lack of positive direction in life.

## Social

- The failure of others to accept that you are ill

- A lack of understanding and support from others

- Needing to prove all the time that you are unwell

- Pressure from others to function normally

- Overprotectiveness by others who do everything for you

- Work stress making it difficult to return to a job.

# Different factors may be important in different people

Careful assessment suggests that people may continue to have CFS/ME for different reasons. In some people, inactivity is an important factor in making them fatigued; in others, it is clearly not. In others, disturbances of sleep seem to be important, and in yet others depression plays a role.

Consequently it is important to treat patients with CFS/ME as individuals and not to assume that the same treatment will work for all of them. The self-help programme we describe has many different parts. You are likely to find that some of these are more helpful to you than others. It may be sensible for you to consider which of the factors we have outlined could be important in perpetuating **your** illness.

## How do these factors interact to perpetuate illness?

The illness-perpetuating factors we have discussed may interact to form vicious circles. We list some examples of these, with suggestions of how they can be broken:

◆ Your sleep is unrefreshing and fragmented. You feel tired. Because you feel so tired you tend to sleep during the day. You are also less active. Doing less and sleeping in the daytime tend to worsen the quality of your night-time sleep. And so on.

   *Advice*—improving the timing and quality of your sleep can help you feel better.

◆ If the changes in brain function make you more easily fatigued, you will be likely to reduce your level of activity, but you may keep making attempts to go on being active—and each time you try you only seem to make yourself feel terrible. You understandably feel that activity is best avoided. A lower level of activity may perpetuate the brain changes that cause fatigue. And so on.

   *Advice*—a very gradual increase in activity seems to reverse the changes in brain function and to help you do more and feel better.

◆ If you are unable to do what you did before you will lack a sense of achievement and may become depressed. Depression makes you more fatigued. Fatigue makes you able to do less. And so on.

   *Advice*—effective treatment of depression can help you do more and feel better.

◆ Stress probably worsens the brain malfunction of CFS/ME. Being unwell is in itself very stressful. This is especially the case if others do not believe that you are really ill. You will probably feel that you should be doing more—and may even doubt your own symptoms. You may try to do what you did before and be unable to sustain it—or simply feel you are letting people down. All these things add to your stress and worsen the symptoms. And so on.

   *Advice*—stress management can help you feel better.

# Targeting treatment

Treatment is aimed at identifying and overcoming illness-perpetuating factors. Identifying any of the vicious circles we have mentioned and finding ways of breaking them will give your body a chance to recover naturally. You might like to trace examples of the vicious circles outlined in the figure below.

Thinking and emotions, behaviour, and physiology all interact with one another. A change in any one can have an effect on the other three. Social factors can also have effects. It can therefore be helpful to think about how all of these things could be influencing you and your illness (and perhaps producing some of the vicious circles we have talked about). Once you have identified what applies to you, you could decide how you could break the circles.

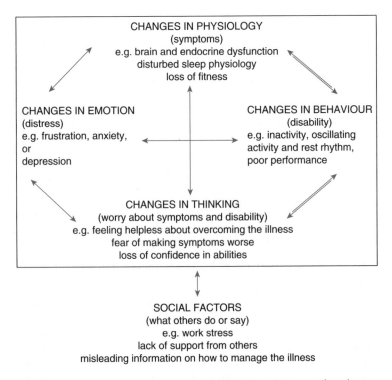

**Figure 7.1** How the factors that can perpetuate CFS/ME can interact and produce vicious circles.

It is unlikely that there is one single cause for CFS/ME. None has been found so far. It may be more useful to look at the three Ps—Predisposing (what makes a person vulnerable), Precipitating (what triggers the illness), and Perpetuating (what keeps the illness going) factors. The perpetuating factors could be physical, psychological, or social—and are often probably a mixture of all three. The trick is to identify those which are important in any particular case and to work towards overcoming these barriers to recovery.

# 8

# What is the best treatment?

 **Key points**

- Many drugs have been tried as treatments for CFS/ME without much success

- Even if a drug is found that could cure CFS/ME, the process of getting a new drug licensed takes many years and it wouldn't be available for some time. So don't put your life on hold waiting for a drug cure

- The best option seems to be the self-help techniques outlined in Section 2

- People do get better from CFS/ME

Many treatments have been tried for CFS/ME. The bad news is that at the present time there is no cure for CFS/ME; the good news is that there is a lot that can be done to manage the illness and speed recovery.

## Research into treatments (clinical trials)

It is important to understand that before a treatment can be recommended it must have been properly tested. The 'gold standard' of such tests is a randomized controlled trial (RCT). In an RCT, patients are allocated randomly to one of two groups; one is given the new treatment and the other is given another treatment (sometimes a placebo or inactive pill, sometimes the current usual care). A comparison group is needed because patients tend to get better anyhow, especially if they are in a trial. As many as a third of patients receiving the placebo treatment tend to report an improvement, so if the new treatment is effective it needs to be substantially better than that.

Allocating patients randomly makes sure that the patients in both groups are similar to start with—both in ways that can be measured and in other ways that might not be obvious. This means that the differences between groups will be due only to the difference in treatment.

RCTs are often done 'blind'. That means that neither the patient nor the doctor giving the treatment is told which treatment a particular patient has received. This is to prevent the effect of the doctors' enthusiasm for the new treatment influencing how they rate the patients' improvement.

A good trial should be as large as possible (a minimum of 50 people and preferably hundreds). This ensures that it includes a wide range of patients and minimizes the risk that any difference (or lack of difference) observed in the effect of the treatments was simply due to chance.

As with all scientific research, it is also important that an RCT is repeated in a different centre, and that similar results are obtained, before we can be certain that any apparent benefit from the new treatment is real.

Finally, the long-term effects of the treatment should be monitored to see how long the benefit lasts for and to ensure that no harmful effects become apparent that were not revealed in the short-term trials.

Any new drug treatment for CFS/ME would have to go through this process before it could be licensed. This is likely to take years. This means that even if a new drug were found very soon, it would not be generally available for some time.

# Choosing a treatment

Having described how treatments have to be tested and what sort of evidence you need to look for, we will now look at a number of treatments that have been proposed for CFS/ME and outline the evidence for their effectiveness.

## No treatment—wait and see

Before considering any treatment, it is worth considering whether it is better to do nothing—simply to wait and see. The advantages of doing this are that no money would be wasted and no adverse treatment effects suffered. The disadvantage is that you would not receive the potential advantage of more active approaches. Whilst for some illnesses a wait-and-see approach is often appropriate, we are concerned that too many people with CFS/ME have accepted this without being aware of the alternatives. These are discussed below.

## Drug treatments

Drugs may be prescribed either to ease a particular symptom or in the hope of dealing with what might be the underlying cause of the condition. As new research findings emerge, so new treatments based on them are tried. So far none of the drug treatments has shown much overall success, although some of them have been reported as having limited benefits for some patients.

### Antiviral drugs

As so many patients report that their illness began with a viral infection and some of the symptoms feel 'viral', this seems a reasonable area for treatment. However trials of antiviral drugs have not been encouraging.

### Drugs to help the immune system

Various drugs acting on the immune system have been tried, but without much success. Other drugs designed to stimulate the immune system, such as Ampligen, are being evaluated and may offer some benefit. However, they are expensive and not yet licensed for use in CFS/ME. They cannot be recommended.

### Drugs to treat low blood pressure

Drugs have been used to treat this condition in patients who have been proved to have it. They may help, but only for those patients with the problem of low blood pressure.

### Cortisol

As we mentioned earlier, research has suggested that some CFS/ME patients have a lower level of cortisol than normal (as opposed to those suffering from depression who often have a higher level), which may perhaps be something to do with the HPA axis not functioning quite normally. This has prompted trials of cortisol as a drug (in the form of hydrocortisone). The results are somewhat mixed, and the serious hazards from taking these steroid drugs long-term outweigh any benefits. At present this treatment cannot be recommended.

### Other hormones and mineral supplements

We are aware that some practitioners advocate a variety of hormones and mineral supplements as treatments for CFS. There is, however, no evidence for the effectiveness of these, and we recommend that they are avoided.

### Antidepressants

The word antidepressant is used as an 'umbrella term' for a group of drugs. One of the actions of these drugs is to improve depressed mood. These drugs also have widespread actions on the functioning of the nervous system, and affect pain, sleep, and appetite as well as mood. It may be more accurate to call them 'brain tonics' rather than antidepressants.

Given that there is now a consensus that the symptoms of CFS/ME are most likely to originate in malfunctioning of the central nervous system, these broad-spectrum 'brain tonics' are possible treatments. There is some (but only limited) evidence that they are effective for CFS/ME. However, they are useful for particular symptoms. Disturbed or unrefreshing sleep can be helped by one of the sedative antidepressants such as amitriptyline (Tryptizol or Elavil) or trazodone (Molipaxin or Desyrel). These drugs can also help with pain. The newer SSRI drugs such as fluoxetine (Prozac) are good for mood but less effective in improving sleep and reducing pain.

If your mood is low and your doctor suspects that you may be depressed, it is worth trying an antidepressant drug. Depression is something that can and should be treated. Having CFS/ME is bad enough without being depressed as well. We talk about this and antidepressants in general in more detail in Chapter 22.

### Analgesics

Pain can be a distressing symptom of CFS/ME, and may respond to analgesics. Painkillers are better used from time to time rather than on a regular basis. You may also benefit from a low dose of a suitable antidepressant, which can be used regularly. We talk about the pros and cons of various analgesics and other ways of managing pain in Chapter 17.

### Sedatives

If you have difficulty getting to sleep or if you wake often during the night it may be tempting to ask your doctor to prescribe a sedative. Such drugs may be helpful if used for just a short time, but, unlike antidepressants, they can produce problems if used for longer. Some of these drugs can be addictive and also become less effective over time. Again a sedative antidepressant may help. We talk about other ways of managing sleep problems in Chapter 15.

### Complementary/alternative therapies

Many people with CFS/ME make use of these therapies. We go into the subject in more detail in Chapter 31. They range from the well-established complementary therapies that your own doctor might suggest, to some alternative therapies that have no scientific basis and which could be dangerous. Many of the alternative therapies involve vitamin or mineral supplements or the use of herbal remedies. However, there is very little evidence that these are necessary or do any good.

If you find something that is helpful to you in some way, then use it. But do be careful. All active treatments—whether complementary, alternative, or conventional—have risks and side effects. Your recovery is probably more likely to depend on what you do for yourself than on any specific therapy you receive.

## Non-drug treatments

So far attempts to identify a drug to treat CFS/ME have had very limited success. However, research into non-drug treatments has produced rather more encouraging results. Some of these treatments have been shown to be a considerable help to patients with CFS/ME.

This seems like a good time to bring up the subject of a referral to a psychologist or to a psychiatrist, as such therapies are often given by them. Some people with CFS/ME feel deeply affronted if their doctor suggests such a referral. They may take it to mean that their doctor does not believe that they have a real illness or may resent the suggestion that emotional problems are the cause. Such feelings are understandable, but if you can overcome them you may find that the referral is helpful to you, particularly if the psychologist or psychiatrist is knowledgeable about CFS/ME.

- Psychologists and psychiatrists are able to give their patients much more time than a busy family doctor can do. For many of the people we have talked with, this was their first opportunity to tell their whole story and discuss **all** their problems. You might find this extremely helpful.

- Any illness is likely to produce some emotional problems. Talking these over with someone who understands them can make them easier to deal with.

- Depression can be a real, if understandable, problem for people with CFS/ME. Although most cases of depression are treated very successfully by family doctors, psychiatrists are more experienced in the treatment of severe depression. They may also be more knowledgeable about tailoring a treatment to suit an individual.

- A psychiatrist can often provide the gateway to the therapies such as CBT (cognitive behaviour therapy) and GET (graded exercise therapy) that we discuss next.

Not all psychiatrists or psychologists will be naturally sympathetic to the patient with CFS/ME, but there are strategies to get the best from your doctors (this topic is discussed further in Chapter 26).

### Cognitive–behavioural therapy (CBT), graded exercise therapy (GET), and adaptive pacing therapy (APT)

These are important non-drug treatments used for CFS/ME. All involve therapists and patients meeting regularly to discuss the illness and how best to manage it. There is good evidence from more than one randomized trial for the effectiveness of CBT and GET in patients with CFS/ME. Pacing or adaptive pacing therapy is widely advocated, but not yet well evaluated. We talk about these therapies in much more detail in Chapter 32.

These treatments are currently being compared with medical care alone in a large UK Medical Research Council-funded randomized clinical trial called PACE (www.pacetrial.org). The results of this trial should be available in 2010.

### Other non-drug treatments: 'reverse' and 'lightening' therapy

In recent years, many new non-drug treatments for CFS/ME have been proposed. Reverse therapy and lightening therapy are just two. Like CBT they aim to aid recovery by changing how patients think about their illness. It is presumed that changed thinking changes brain function. Whilst some patients have found these treatments helpful, others have not and have indeed found them to be harmful. They have not been evaluated in randomized trials so their true effectiveness (and potential for harm) cannot be reliably predicted. They are also privately provided and can be expensive. For these reasons, we cannot recommend them.

# Do people get better from CFS/ME?

Yes they do. Most people tend to improve, but it may take time. If you have CFS/ME you are most likely to get better if you use the self-help techniques outlined in Section 2 or if you pursue a treatment of proven benefit such as CBT or GET. In trials, about two-thirds of patients who have these treatments are much improved a year later compared with one-third of those who have only medical care. In most, the benefits will last. Whilst most of these patients get back to a normal life, we have noted that many choose a different, less pressurized occupation.

Doctors cannot simply prescribe a drug that will cure CFS/ME. Whilst it is possible that this situation may change, it is not likely to happen in the near future. Putting your life on hold waiting for a miracle drug is therefore not a good idea. You do have other options. Probably the best option today is to work on positively managing your symptoms. You can do this using the self-help techniques we talk about in Section 2. These self-help techniques may be easier to do if you have help from a person or therapist who can guide you. However, there is much you can do yourself by simply using this book. People do get better from CFS/ME, and this is most likely to happen if you manage your illness as described in this book.

# 9

# Some myths about CFS/ME

## 🡢 Key points

♦ There are many incorrect or only partially correct things said and written about CFS/ME

♦ Do not let these 'myths' distract or discourage you from managing your illness sensibly yourself

Before reading this book you have probably heard or read a variety of things about CFS or ME. Some of these things may have been only partially correct or, worse still, not true at all. Some of these 'myths' may get in the way of you effectively managing your illness. Here are some of the 'ME myths' we have heard about:

♦ *The only treatment for CFS/ME is rest, rest, and more rest.* This is very far from the truth. Everybody needs good-quality rest, and people with CFS/ME are no exception. However, research has shown that too much rest is not good for anyone. Like too much food, it has long-term harmful effects. Rest is best balanced with regular daily activity. For people with CFS/ME, the amount of activity may initially need to be small and only increased gradually.

♦ *People with CFS/ME should never take antibiotics.* Indiscriminate use of antibiotics for any ailment is not good for anyone. However, there is no reason to avoid them when needed. For instance, if you developed an abscess under a tooth, that would certainly be an appropriate time for antibiotic treatment.

♦ *Anaesthetics are bad for people with CFS/ME.* This is often said, but it is based on no real evidence. Any operation is likely to be tiring and stressful, especially if you are feeling ill to start with, but there is no good evidence that the anaesthetic is more harmful if you have CFS/ME. Do not allow yourself to be put off having essential treatment.

◆ *If you have CFS/ME, you have a problem with Candida overgrowth in your intestines.* There is no good evidence for this idea. It is a myth.

◆ *If you are not trying alternative therapies you are not really trying to get better.* If you try the self-help techniques we advocate, you will certainly be doing your best. (What is more, they will cost you very much less.) There is no alternative therapy of proven effectiveness in CFS/ME—whatever people may claim.

◆ *You should be using large amounts of dietary supplements.* Again, this is something that has not been proved by proper research. It is a myth.

◆ *You should have any dental fillings containing mercury amalgam removed.* There is little evidence that mercury amalgam fillings have much effect on anyone. There is no good evidence that they cause CFS/ME. The process of removal could be very expensive, potentially hazardous, and certainly would be very stressful and tiring. It would probably do you much more harm than good.

◆ *Until a drug cure is found, there is nothing that can be done to help a person with CFS/ME.* Although there is as yet no drug therapy to cure the condition, research has clearly shown that the sort of techniques described in this book can make a difference to your well-being. Such techniques can be even more effective if practised with the help of a knowledgeable therapist.

◆ *CBT and GET are harmful for people with CFS/ME.* They are not harmful if properly given. They are simply ways of helping people with CFS/ME to increase activity **at their own pace**. Forced increases in activity are not part of proper GET or CBT. Most patients with CFS/ME who have tried and persevered with CBT and GET have been able to do more as a result. As with all active treatments, there is a risk of side effects, and a small number of patients who have been treated with GET and CBT report feeling worse afterwards. There is, however, no evidence that they have been harmed. Why not read Chapter 32 in which we describe what is actually involved in CBT and GET treatments for CFS/ME and then you can judge for yourself?

It is not only fellow sufferers who can spread myths about CFS/ME. Doctors can do so too. Some medical recommendations reported back to us by patients are also myths:

◆ *CFS/ME is not a real illness. It is all in your mind.* CFS/ME **is** a real illness and involves both the body **and** the mind.

- *You should push yourself through it.* Cautious increases in activity after stabilizing your level of activity can be helpful; rushing into increased activity is generally not.

- *You need exercise therapy. Go to your local gym and get to work.* **Graded** exercise therapy is something very different from that. It involves cautious and structured increases in activity.

- *You are just depressed.* It is possible that you are depressed. 'Just' is hardly an appropriate word. Depression is serious and can cause physical symptoms. You can be depressed and also suffering from CFS/ME.

- *There is nothing that can be done to help with CFS/ME. You will just have to wait for a natural recovery.* You can do a lot to help yourself in the process of recovery. You do not have wait helplessly.

As you get more experienced in managing your condition, you will be more able to distinguish myths from reality on the basis of your own experience. Do not let myths discourage you from gathering more insight into your illness by trying out the self-help techniques that we discuss in the next section.

# 10

# Summary

As you can see from all we have written in this section, there is a shortage of real facts about CFS/ME and also about some of the associated conditions. No one is certain exactly what causes these illnesses. There is no diagnostic test for them and there is no medical treatment that has been proved to help everyone. However, we do know quite a lot about barriers to recovery from CFS/ME and how to overcome them. There is a great deal that people who suffer from these illnesses can do to help themselves. We will talk about this in the next section of the book. To sum up what is **known** about the best way of dealing with CFS/ME:

* Do not put your life on hold waiting for the 'magic bullet' medical treatment. You may wait a long time. You also do not have to wait to be **made** well—instead you can concentrate on all the things that will help you **get** well.

* Do not neglect treatable aspects of your illness. For instance, if you suffer from depression, get treatment for that. If you have severe pain, consider the careful use of painkillers. Anything that reduces the overall burden on you will be helpful.

* Get good rest but also keep active. Try to get your sleep and activity into a comfortable and regular pattern.

* Once you have stabilized your daily routine, try to expand it by very gradual increases toward planned targets.

* Managing yourself and your illness is the key to success.

In the next section of the book we describe what you can do to manage your illness. Do read it with an open mind. What we suggest is based on research and on years of experience of listening to and advising people with CFS/ME. You have nothing to lose by trying out these techniques, and we believe that you have a lot to gain.

# Section 2

# The idea of helping yourself

# 11

# Introduction to self-help

> ### ➜ Key points
>
> ◆ Though there is not yet a proven medical cure for CFS/ME, there is a great deal you can do to help yourself

The fact that there is as yet no single identified cause or proven medical cure for CFS/ME does **not** mean that there is nothing that can be done about the condition. For a start, your doctor may be able to help you with symptom relief and perhaps refer you to other health professionals who can assist you in your quest for improvement.

More importantly though, there is a great deal that you can do to help yourself. Our bodies are very good at healing themselves if we give them a chance. We now know quite a lot about what you can do to help (or hinder) your body's natural healing (based on both research evidence and clinical experience). This section of the book will outline all the things that will help, both to make you feel better and to give you the best chance of being able to regain a normal life.

We are going to start by looking at what you can do in an effective way to manage your life and your illness by adopting what might be called 'health-promoting behaviours'. Later we will look at how your emotions can have an effect on your condition. Finally, we will suggest some practical ideas about ways in which you could make your life easier or more pleasurable, which would also be an aid to improvement. You might also read our other book *Living with a Long-Term Illness: The Facts* published by Oxford Uuniversity Press in 2006, which covers these topics in more detail.

As you read through this section, you may feel that it is a bit daunting. What we suggest may seem to require too much discipline and too many changes in the ways you currently manage your life and your illness. Most people have these reservations at first, but find that it gets easier as they persevere and that the benefits make the discipline and changes worthwhile.

It will certainly make a difference if you can get support from those around you—people such as a partner, family, or friends—by helping them understand what you are doing and why. Perhaps you could get them to read this section of the book if not all of it.

## How to do it

Depending on where you live, you may be able to attend one of the specialist clinics that offer help and advice for people with CFS/ME. If you do not have access to one of these, this section will outline what such a service might advise so that you can treat yourself. It will help if you can find someone knowledgeable who can support you in what you are doing. Many doctors, occupational therapists, psychologists, and counsellors are able to do this. Alternatively, you might have someone close to you who could give you help and encouragement. However, even if you have no help, it is quite possible to do it on your own.

## When to start

The earlier in your illness that you can begin this active illness management the better, but there is no reason to assume that if you have been ill for some time this sort of thing is not for you. We know of many people who have been ill for a long time who have made significant improvement when they changed the way they were managing their illness. Even if you are very severely ill, there is a possibility of improvement, though it may be a very long slow process. Patience and discipline are going to be important (sorry about that!).

# 12

# Balancing rest and activity

**➲ Key points**

◆ 'Pacing'—balancing rest and activity in a consistent way—is one of the most important tools in a self-help programme

◆ Stopping any activity in good time, before you get too tired, is important. Don't be overambitious

◆ Good-quality rest between bouts of activity will help you feel less ill

Balancing rest and activity is one of the most important things that you can do to help yourself. Although we can describe general principles, you will need to work out a personalized 'programme' of rest and activity to suit you and the way you are now. After all, **you** are the expert on **you**.

## The 'roller coaster'

Too many people with CFS/ME live on a roller coaster, alternating bursts of activity with periods of rest. They do too much one day, feel much worse as a result, and are then able to do much less for the next day or two. After resting during this time they wake up feeling much better and immediately try to catch up, do too much, and crash again. This does not help them to recover and usually adds to their feelings of frustration. Many people with this pattern of activity end up being able to do less in total because the times when they are active are outweighed by the times when they can do so little. It is often said that CFS/ME is a very fluctuating condition; in our experience, it is sometimes the way that the person with CFS/ME copes that fluctuates, leading to episodic exacerbation of symptoms. Pacing is a way of avoiding this problem.

# Pacing

'Pacing' means maintaining a steady level of activity overall by balancing periods of activity, both physical and mental, with periods of good-quality rest. Your aim should be to work out how much you can do and stop **before** you get exhausted. Getting a bit tired will not do you any harm, but getting exhausted on a regular basis is not helpful. The best idea is to start at a level well within your capacity, even if that means doing rather less to begin with. The principles of pacing will help you whatever your level of activity. You are likely to find that stopping while you are still only a bit tired, rather than keeping going until you are exhausted, will mean that you need much shorter periods of rest to recover from the exertion. Balancing activity and rest is also likely to help you feel better.

Mental activity can be as tiring as physical activity, so something like sitting watching television does not count as real rest. Try to alternate using your body and using your mind, with intervals of proper rest between each activity.

Pacing may mean changing your way of life considerably and accepting that you often have to stop something before you have finished it, take a break for a rest, and then come back to it later. Pacing requires discipline. In Chapter 20 we look at what can make achieving that discipline more difficult—'what gets in the way of being sensible'. Wait until you have read that chapter before you decide that it is all too difficult for you. In Chapter 27 we explain 'budgeting' your energy expenditure, which can also help.

# Keeping an activity diary

It may help if you keep a brief diary for a **few** weeks in which you record your activity and how you feel. After you have kept a record for a while, you will probably be able to spot patterns such as the swings between doing too much, feeling unwell, and then doing little. You will need to look for patterns over more than a single day as it is typical of CFS/ME that the effects of getting too tired may not show up until the next day or even the day after. You need to anticipate this. You can use the information from this diary to help you to plan out a 'programme' of balanced rest and activity. A structure to your day, with targets set and achieved (however small they may need to be), will help give you back a sense of control in your life. You will find details of such a diary in Appendix 2.

# Pleasure and satisfaction

When you are planning your programme, it is important to include at least some activities that give you pleasure or satisfaction. Pleasure is one of the things that is really good for your body and for your spirit. It is so easy to believe that, because you have got CFS/ME and cannot do all the things you once could, you cannot enjoy yourself. That is not necessarily so. It is worth exploring other ways of enjoying yourself that fit in with your present circumstances. We talk more about this in Chapter 27.

## Rewards

Many people find it easier to stick to a pacing programme if they do not make it too rigid and if they give themselves rewards for sticking to their plan.

> Jake found that he could be much more successful in his pacing if he gave himself a treat at the end of a week in which he had managed to stay disciplined. He allowed himself a long-distance call to a good friend, partly as a reward and partly to report how well he had done.

## Where are you now?

Accept where you are now. What can you comfortably do now (and not just on a good day) and then repeat on the next day? Be honest with yourself. This is your starting point. We are often asked 'How long should my periods of activity be?'. Each person is different, so there is no absolute rule. Your activity diary should help you decide what is an appropriate period and what is 'going on too long' for each activity. If in doubt, start low.

## Be consistent

Your 'programme' should be something you can keep up in a **consistent** way. Consistency really is vital even though it may mean that, for a while, you may have to do rather less. However, many people are surprised to find that by spreading out their activities (over the day and over the week) they end up being able to do rather more.

> Sue used to do her housework in one burst in the morning, only stopping when she was completely exhausted. The rest of the day she felt very ill as well as frustrated by not having been able to achieve all she wanted. Then she tried the experiment of limiting herself to 15 minute chunks of activity. Between these chunks she sat down, relaxed, and had a rest. At the end of the first week she was astonished to find that she had achieved more and yet was not feeling so tired and ill.

You may find that it takes some time to adjust to this new way of doing things. You probably will not get it right immediately and will need to keep working at it. Most people find it takes time to change. You do not need to be too rigid about your programme either. There are bound to be times when things outside your control get in the way. Do not worry about that; just come back to the programme again as soon as you can.

## Make increases gradually

Later on you are likely to find that it can be possible to increase the amount you do, either by making your periods of activity just a little longer or by doing things in short periods more often during the day. However, it is vital that when you make these sort of changes you do it in a gradual way; 'go slow'. We talk more about this in Chapter 19.

Sticking to a consistent pattern of physical and mental activities, both during the day and during the week, with intervals of rest between activities is one of the best things you can do to help yourself. Plan out a programme for yourself and make sure that it includes things that give you pleasure or satisfaction, as well as the necessary chores. This consistent programme could well reduce some of your symptoms and start you on the path towards improvement. Remember, 'start low and go slow'.

# 13

# Relaxation and calm breathing

> ## ➲ Key points
>
> ◆ Being able to relax both your body and your mind is a skill most people need to learn and to practise regularly
>
> ◆ Regular periods of relaxation and calm breathing will help you feel better and get better quality rest

Relaxation is one of those words that mean different things to different people. What we mean in this context is not just 'taking it easy'. We mean letting go of physical tension in all your muscles.

Deep physical relaxation and calm breathing are both things that will help your body. In the previous chapter we talked about periods of good-quality rest between activities. You will rest much better if all your muscles are relaxed. It may take time and practice to learn how to do this. There are tapes and books available that can help you in this (you will find some suggestions in Appendix 3), but you can start it on your own.

## When and where

Choose a time when you are not going to be disturbed and get yourself really comfortable, whether lying down or sitting in a chair that supports your neck and arms, in dim light if you prefer.

## Relax your muscles

Some people find that if they first tighten up the part they want to relax it helps them to recognize the difference between being tense and being relaxed.

Start by taking a few calm, slow breaths. Now think about one hand. Tighten it up into a clenched fist for a moment and then let it go. Feel the difference between tight and loose. Think about your hand, wrist, and arm getting warmer and heavier. If someone were to take hold of your cuff and lift your wrist, you would not help them by using your arm muscles and when they let go your hand would flop down again. Move round your body letting go of the tension in all your muscle groups in the same way. Your shoulders and neck are an important area to concentrate on. Think about your face too. If you are frowning or your teeth are clenched, it is much more difficult to relax. Work towards a calm, peaceful expression. Tensing up a muscle before relaxing it is not necessary all the time, but it helps when you are first learning how to relax.

## Relax your breathing

Calm breathing is important. Some people with CFS/ME breathe rapidly or erratically, particularly if they are feeling anxious or panicky. Learning good breathing techniques and practising them regularly will really help. Your aim should be to breathe slowly and deeply—letting your ribs and your diaphragm do the work, rather than just the top of your chest. You could ask for help from your doctor or a physiotherapist if you find this difficult.

## Relax your mind

Your relaxation periods are **not** times for thinking hard or for worrying. Try to switch off from anxious or unhappy thoughts by thinking about something else, something peaceful and happy. Trying to make your mind a blank does not work. Some people find it helps if they visualize a special place, a sanctuary all their own, concentrating on all the details of sight, sound, smell, etc. Others find the techniques of meditation extremely helpful in giving them a period of calmness and rest. Experiment with what works for you.

## After relaxing

When you come to the end of your relaxation period, do not leap up immediately. Give yourself a little time to take a few deep breaths and to stretch a little. Think about how a cat stretches before it gets up.

## Practise

Do not feel that you have to master this skill right away. Spend time on it and practise it regularly. As you get better at it, you will find that you can switch it on whenever you need it—and not necessarily just while lying down. Periods of relaxation and calm breathing during the day may help to reduce pain and the 'flu-like' feelings. It is certainly one of the things that will help you get to sleep and cope with periods of wakefulness during the night. It is also a technique that will help you deal better with stress.

## Possible problems

To begin with, you may find that you do not enjoy relaxation or find it comfortable. Some people tell us that they notice pain or fatigue more when they are not being distracted from it by activity. (This does not mean that the symptoms **are** worse—just that they are more noticeable.) If you have been in the habit of keeping yourself busy, switching off may make you feel a little guilty at first. Remind yourself that you need to do this to get well; it will get easier and more enjoyable with practice.

Being able to relax both your body and your mind is a skill that many people need to learn and to practise. Regular periods of relaxation will help you to feel better and get better quality rest.

# 14

# Appropriate exercise

➡ **Key points**

◆ Too much rest is not good for anyone. Keeping your body moving will avoid the dangers of getting out of condition. Bodies are designed to move

◆ To start, aim for small, planned amounts of exercise that do not leave you too tired

◆ Once you have settled to a stable amount of exercise you can plan for a very gradual increase

## Rest

You may well have found that doing nothing for a day or two reduces your symptoms. Understandably, therefore, you may have decided that more rest is the answer. However, though we all need reasonable periods of good-quality rest, too much rest also has bad effects. It leads to muscle weakness, stiff joints, poor circulation with postural hypotension (loss of blood pressure control causing dizziness on standing up), and back problems. It also causes loss of motivation and poor concentration, and in the long term more fatigue. Research for the American space programme found that prolonged rest—even for periods as short as 2 weeks—can cause these changes, even in fit young people.

The periods of relaxation that we discussed in the previous chapter are **not** the same as prolonged rest. Short periods during which you relax your body and mind are very beneficial; **prolonged** rest (lasting days and weeks) is not.

# Are you suffering from the effects of inactivity?

**Some** of the problems and symptoms you are experiencing now could be because of being inactive since you became ill. This is sometimes called de-conditioning. (We do not mean by this that de-conditioning is the only reason you are still ill.) For instance, spending a lot of time lying in bed can make you feel weak and worsen back pain. Bodies are made to move. It really will help your body if you can keep it moving, even if all you can manage is a small amount at intervals during the day. Little and often works well. Try to build appropriate periods of physical activity into your 'pacing programme'. If you are uncertain where to start, you could ask for a fitness assessment from a physiotherapist, who would be able to plan out an exercise programme appropriate for the way you are now.

# Getting fitter

Try not to be overambitious. Forget what you used to be able to do before you were ill. You can only start from where you are now. Just concentrate on what suits your body **now** and work out what you can do comfortably and for how long. Warm up with gentle stretches and stop when you have completed what you planned. Don't carry on until you feel too tired to continue. A small amount done regularly is going to do you much more good than doing too much one day and being too tired to do anything the next day.

Here are some suggestions about how you can help yourself:

♦   *Bending and stretching exercises*—joints that are not used get stiff, muscles that are not used can get shorter and weaker, so very gentle exercises will help avoid problems. Start very gradually. You can do gentle exercises even while lying down.

♦   *Walking*—this is one of the best forms of exercise, even if you can only manage a small amount. Two short walks morning and afternoon are better than one longer one that leaves you exhausted. You will probably find that by splitting your walks into smaller chunks you will be able to walk further in total. You may only be able to manage a few paces at first, but even that will be a good start.

♦   *Swimming and cycling*—if your condition allows it, these are both good forms of exercise if done gently and in moderation. Pace yourself carefully, always stopping before you get too tired.

◆ *Posture*—if you are feeling tired and weak, it is very tempting to slouch or sit in a slumped position. Think tall!! Good posture is much kinder to your body.

Once you have achieved a level of exercise that you can do in a consistent way, you can begin the process of increasing it very gradually. This is something we discuss in more detail in Chapter 19.

Keeping your body moving will help avoid the dangers of getting out of condition and will keep you in the best shape possible. Bodies are made to move. Aim for small planned amounts, done regularly, that do not leave you too tired. Once you have found a stable level of exercise that you can tolerate, the next step is to plan a gradual increase.

# 15

# Improving your sleep

➡ **Key points**

♦ Many people with CFS/ME have problems with their sleep

♦ Self-help techniques to aid sleep can make a real difference

♦ Try to avoid worrying at night time. Give yourself a 'worry time' during the day

♦ The use of sedatives on a regular basis is best avoided

People with CFS/ME often find that their sleep pattern has changed. At the beginning of their illness they sometimes sleep much more. Later on they may find that they have difficulty getting to sleep or that they may wake during the night. Often, even if they have slept, they still wake up feeling tired. Good-quality sleep, at normal times, is something we all need, so it is worth looking at all the ways that you can get back to this.

## Getting to sleep

You can experiment with all the things that help you get to sleep, such as establishing a calm routine that leads up to bedtime and relaxing when you get to bed. The period just before sleep is **not** the time for thinking about problems—which will make it much harder for you to settle down. Many people find it helpful to set up a specific 'worry time' earlier in the day. If you find that you tend to worry about some problem while you are trying to get to sleep, tell yourself that you will think about that problem tomorrow during your worry time. It is wise to avoid alcohol and caffeine-containing drinks for a couple of hours before bedtime—they may make it harder to get to sleep.

# Getting back to sleep if you wake in the night

If you wake during the night, try to stay calm and relaxed. Build up a collection of gentle, pleasant things to occupy your mind. That way you will still be getting rest and you are more likely to fall asleep again. Relaxation techniques (as in Chapter 13) will help you get the most rest possible while you are awake.

Worrying about not sleeping is almost guaranteed to make it much harder to get back to sleep. If you really cannot sleep, get up and do something else such as reading or listening to music until you begin to feel sleepy again. Then go back to bed—and to sleep!

# Establishing a pattern

You need to establish regular times for going to bed and for waking. Research into body rhythms in people with CFS/ME has shown how important this is. Many people have noticed the similarity between the symptoms of CFS/ME and those of 'jet lag'.

You may need to re-establish such a regular pattern. This will mean avoiding sleeping at other times. If you have slept badly during the night, it is very tempting to sleep longer in the morning, but this is not a good idea. The sleep patterns of some people with CFS/ME can get chaotic, even going as far as sleeping most of the day and being awake most of the night. This makes it difficult to take part in normal social activity and can worsen the illness by disrupting your body rhythms. You may need to use an alarm clock or a timed radio to help you wake at a regular time. You can always rest later in the day if you need it.

If you are feeling very tired, it may seem reasonable to have naps during the day. This may be the right thing for you, but not if it makes it more difficult to get to sleep at night. If you want a daytime nap (and if it will fit into your schedule) try to have it at a regular time (like a 'siesta' after lunch). Experiment to see what works best for you.

# Using sedatives

If these simple 'sleep hygiene' methods are not enough, you might want to consider taking one of the several types of sedative medicine. The most commonly prescribed ones are benzodiazepines such as temazepam. These are safe and effective but can interfere with the quality of sleep and, if used for long periods, can also be addictive. It is better to avoid using sleeping pills on a regular basis if you can, and to establish a natural pattern. However, you could talk to your doctor about using them for a limited period.

An alternative to sleeping pills is to take a low dose of a sedative 'antidepressant' drug such as amitriptyline (Tryptizol or Elavil) or trazodone (Molipaxin or Desyrel) an hour or two before you go to bed. These drugs are not just prescribed to help mood; they have a lot of useful effects for improving sleep and helping with pain. At this low dosage they are very unlikely to have any unpleasant side effects, and they are not addictive.

> Improving your sleep pattern is an important part of your overall strategy for helping your body to recover. It is worth experimenting to find what helps. Try to stay relaxed if you do find it difficult to go to sleep or if you wake during the night. Worrying about not sleeping will only make things worse.

# 16

# Getting the best from your food

## ➡ Key points

♦ A good, well-balanced diet with meals at regular times is an important part of looking after yourself. Food is something you should enjoy

♦ Massive supplements of minerals and vitamins are not necessary for people with CFS/ME

If you are feeling very tired and unwell it can be all too easy to neglect yourself, by going for easy meals and eating at odd hours. Regular, good-quality meals should be part of your plan for giving yourself the best chance of improvement. Try to get back into the habit of having good-quality meals at consistent, normal times—breakfast, lunch, and supper. Some people feel better if they do not go for too long between meals. If you are one of them, then including small, healthy snacks between meals can be a good idea.

## A normal healthy diet

What should you be eating? Basically, what you should be aiming for is a well-balanced diet of good-quality food including all the different food groups. Many people prefer a low-fat, low-sugar diet. However, you should try to include a wide variety of food. The following are generally accepted as part of a healthy diet:

Complex carbohydrates (wholemeal bread rather than white), pulses (beans, lentils, etc.), plenty of fresh fruit, salads, and lightly cooked vegetables, good-quality low-fat protein, milk, and cheeses, eggs, liver (but not if you are pregnant), and oily fish (such as tuna and mackerel).

We are **not** suggesting a special diet for people with CFS/ME—just the sort of good food that makes up a normal healthy diet and which doctors would recommend for anyone. Beware of restrictive diets suggested as treatment—there is no evidence that they help and they may harm you.

## Food supplements

Your aim should be to get all the nourishment you need from what you are eating. You may have read that if you have CFS/ME you should be taking massive supplements of minerals and vitamins. There is no evidence at all that this is necessary. Supplements like these can be very expensive. Nourishment is probably more easily absorbed from food than from pills. It can be dangerous to take too much of some vitamins (such as vitamin A), and for most others our bodies simply excrete what they do not need, so you could end up with most of what you have paid for disappearing down the toilet.

## Alcohol, tea, and coffee

Many people with CFS/ME find that alcohol makes them feel worse. If you are one of them, you may wish to limit your intake or even to cut it out. Other people also choose to reduce the amount of tea, coffee, and cola they drink (all of them contain the stimulant caffeine).

## Weight change

Being overweight or underweight can both be unhelpful to your recovery. If you are taking much less exercise because of your illness and yet are still eating the same amount as before you became ill, it is very easy to put on weight. Comfort eating can also lead to weight gain. Carrying too much weight will only add to your fatigue. Similarly, it is not helpful to lose too much weight. If you have a problem with weight, talk to a doctor or dietician and get advice on a diet that will get you to a sensible weight and keep your weight stable.

Depression can lead to weight loss and to weight gain. Some people who are suffering from depression eat more and some lose their appetite. Some of the drugs that are used to treat depression can have a side effect of increasing appetite and others of reducing it. Discuss this with your doctor if he or she is prescribing an antidepressant for you.

## Tired of cooking (or tired by cooking)?

Eating well does not mean that you have to spend a lot of time cooking. You can get all the nourishment you need from very simple food. For instance, a sandwich made from wholemeal bread, cold meat, or tinned tuna, with a tomato or some fresh fruit and a glass of milk is a perfectly healthy meal. If you are intolerant of certain foods, you would have to plan sensible alternatives.

## Keeping diet and food as normal as possible

One general rule that applies here is that it is better to do things as normally as possible unless there is a **good** reason not to. You do not need to change from your previous eating habits unless they included a lot of junk food or irregular meal times, or if you have a problem with your weight. If so, this might be a good moment to change to a regular, healthy diet which would be something of benefit to you for the rest of your life. Enjoying what you eat is one of the basic pleasures in life, so try to eat healthily and happily.

A good, well-balanced diet with meals at regular times is an important part of looking after yourself and part of your strategy for improvement. Give your body all the nourishment it needs for health and recovery. Supplements of vitamins and minerals are not necessary for most people with CFS/ME. Food is something you should enjoy.

## 17

# Coping with pain

➡ **Key points**

♦ Pain is a common problem for people with CFS/ME

♦ Make sure that your pain is not caused by some other problem

♦ There are ways of coping with pain that can lessen its impact

♦ Painkillers can help, but try to avoid using opiates and drugs containing codeine

For many people, pain is one of the most difficult and distressing symptoms of CFS/ME. We often hear patients say 'I could cope with just being tired. It's the pain that makes life so difficult'. It may be a constant background to your life or it may be intermittent, perhaps made worse by overactivity. Being in pain can be tiring and can often interfere with sleep, so anything you can do to manage your pain—to reduce it or to lessen its impact—will be a help to both your body and your mind. Different people experience different kinds of pain. The most common in CFS/ME are widespread muscle and joint pains, but pain can occur anywhere. We can offer you some suggestions for strategies for managing your own pain, but, as with most of what we suggest, you will have to experiment to find what works for you.

## Check out that it is all due to CFS/ME

Do not assume that every symptom is due to CFS/ME. Discuss this with your family doctor or your consultant. Make sure that other conditions that could cause pain have been considered and treated.

Consider whether some of your pain could be a consequence of lack of activity or poor posture. This is likely to be an added factor if you lead a very sedentary life or spend a lot of time in bed. Muscles that are not used get weaker; joints get stiff like rusty hinges. When they are used they hurt. You could try a minimal exercise routine to stretch and strengthen your muscles and to keep your joints mobile (as in Chapter 14). Good posture may help to prevent some of these problems.

## Relaxation

Pain is made worse by muscle tension. Sometimes the pain is actually caused by it. For instance, some headaches are a result of tension in the neck and shoulders. Try the effect of relaxing in response to pain instead of tightening up against it.

## Distraction

Pain is always more of a problem when we are focusing our attention on it. The more we concentrate on it, the worse it is likely to seem. Distraction is a good technique to help reduce your awareness of your pain, even if you can only keep it up for a few minutes at a time. Any moments of respite are to be welcomed. Once you have got yourself relaxed, try moving on to focusing your awareness on something else. Experiment to find out what works best for you. It could be music or a talking book, or just thinking of something pleasant and relaxing. Sometimes concentrating on a bit of your body that is **not** hurting, even if it is just your little finger, can help.

## Splitting the sensation and the message

This sounds complicated, so let us explain what we mean. Before you became ill, a sudden onset of pain was a danger signal. It could mean that something was going wrong and was often a cause for quite reasonable alarm. However, when pain has been there a long time it is less likely to mean that there is anything dangerous going on. You may well be afraid that pain means that you are getting worse, that you have caused yourself permanent damage or that you have some life-threatening condition. We so often hear patients saying things like 'I know it sounds silly, but could such-and-such a pain mean that I could have heart disease/cancer/a brain tumour . . .?'. You are not alone if you sometimes have thoughts like these. Fear is a distressing and demoralizing emotion, and it is exhausting too. It is important to look at the meanings you give to your pain, and to check their accuracy. You may need to seek a medical opinion to make sure that you are not suffering from a dangerous condition.

After that, the more that you can reduce the feelings of fear and resentment of pain, the easier it will be for you and the better it will be for your body. Fear and anger are stressful, and stress often makes CFS/ME worse. Tension caused by these emotions can make your pain worse. You may need to talk through your feelings of anger and resentment that you are hurting so much. Anything that helps in that way will be good for you and make the pain easier to cope with.

## Other techniques

It is worth trying out all the things that help just a little. Do you hurt less if you are warm? Maybe a hot-water bottle in the right place will help, or an electric blanket in your bed would make a difference. Does a warm bath make you feel better? A bath does not have to be only for washing—you could just relax and enjoy it.

The right kind of massage can sometimes help. You need to experiment to find what works for you. Perhaps you could train a partner or a friend to do massage for you, even if you cannot afford professional sessions.

Some people find that acupuncture can be effective for their particular kind of pain, though the relief may not last.

You may find that visualization can help. Some people can form a picture in their minds of their pain. If you are one of them, you could experiment with trying to change the picture into something less aggressive (like changing an image of a tiger into one of a gentle kitten). If you think of the pain in a colour, you could try changing that colour to something softer and more friendly.

## Painkillers

Like all medicines, painkillers (analgesic medication) have advantages and disadvantages. It is therefore worth trying other strategies for managing pain, such as we have outlined earlier, rather than just relying on drugs. Whilst pain-relieving drugs work well in the short term, in the longer term they can become ineffective and even addictive. There is also evidence that prolonged use of analgesics can make headaches worse. All painkillers have some side effects, and people with CFS/ME may be sensitive to them. However, if you find something that works for you, even if you only use it very infrequently, it can make day-to-day pain easier to manage. You do not have to feel 'I have to bear this for ever'. Almost anything is easier to cope with if you know you could have moments when you could choose not to have to cope. One word of warning—beware that relief from pain doesn't make you lose sight of your pacing programme.

Common analgesic drugs include:

♦ Soluble aspirin or paracetamol (acetaminophen) can sometimes give some relief, but they can cause gastric problems or liver problems if used excessively.

♦ Anti-inflammatory drugs such as ibuprofen (Brufen or Motrin) can sometimes help with pain in muscles and joints, but again may cause gastric problems.

♦ As with sleep problems, a low dose of the so-called antidepressants such as amitriptyline (Tryptizol or Elavil) used on a regular basis can help with pain (whether or not you feel depressed). They are often used in Pain Relief Clinics for a variety of conditions causing pain. They are not addictive.

Opiates and drugs containing codeine are better not used on a regular basis. They can cause constipation and can interfere with sleep. They may be addictive.

---

Pain is a common problem for people with CFS/ME, but there are ways in which you can lessen its impact on you. First make sure that the pain doesn't have another cause. Then use the self-help techniques we have outlined. It is generally better to avoid opiates and drugs including codeine if you can. Experiment with the techniques we have outlined and see what helps you.

# 18

# Difficulties with memory and concentration

> ## ➲ Key points
>
> ◆ Many people with CFS/ME experience difficulties with memory and concentration, especially when they are tired
>
> ◆ This does not indicate any permanent brain damage
>
> ◆ As your condition improves, these problems will get less

One of the symptoms of CFS/ME that can cause great distress and be very worrying is that of difficulties with memory and concentration. This is something that is very often reported by patients. It is quite normal to have these problems. They do **not** mean that there is any permanent brain damage. These problems will get less as your health improves. Research has shown that the degree of difficulty in things such as short-term memory and concentration vary to some extent with your level of fatigue, and with how ill you are feeling. Though these problems can be infuriating (and at times extremely inconvenient), they are not something to fear.

What sort of problems do patients with CFS/ME report? A common one is difficulty reading, not necessarily because of eye problems (though they may be there too) but because it is hard to remember what happened earlier in the book. Another problem is difficulty in finding the right word, or using the wrong word, which can be very disconcerting both for the sufferer and for those around them. Problems with memory mean that we often hear of people going into a room to do something and then finding that they cannot remember what it was. Concentration is often more difficult when you are tired.

# Helping yourself

There is a lot you can do to help yourself, both in propping up a faulty memory and in doing small things to keep your brain active:

◆ Cut down on what you absolutely have to remember. Do not try to remember anything that you could write down.

◆ Use lists; write yourself notes. It can be helpful to use a notebook, or something like a Filofax, so you know where you have made the note—you can waste a lot of time and effort trying to remember on which scrap of paper you wrote the information!

◆ Try to build up rituals and routines to help you remember things—like always putting the car keys in the same place immediately you come into the house.

◆ Give yourself a few moments before you do something to get it clear in your head.

◆ Take time to consider what causes you the greatest difficulty and then think about practical ways to make things easier.

If you have difficulty concentrating, try doing the things that require concentration in much smaller 'bites'. Do a small amount, have a rest, and then come back to it later. Cut out distractions such as noise or conversation. Choose a time of day when concentration seems a little easier to do the demanding tasks. One of the tasks that people with CFS/ME often find difficult and stressful is filling in official forms. Allow yourself to tackle them slowly, perhaps just doing one page or section a day. Forcing yourself to go on until it is finished will be very tiring and will probably mean that you do it much less efficiently. A warning note—putting off the difficult task will often mean that you face a deadline and then need to do it in a hurry. Try to start in good time.

# Keeping in practice

It is also well worth keeping in regular practice with the things you find difficult. If you give up bothering with something because it is difficult, it is likely to get worse because you are out of practice ('use it or lose it'). Your brain needs exercise as much as your body. To give just one example, if you often have difficulty finding the right word, crossword puzzles can be a useful brain exercise. You do not need to do all of a puzzle, but just trying a few clues of the simplest puzzle will keep you in practice at retrieving the right word.

Difficulties with memory and concentration are common in CFS/ME, but they do not indicate permanent damage. Use every technique possible to make life easier for yourself. As your condition improves, these problems will get less. Keep on using your brain, even if it is difficult.

## 19

# A gradual increase in activity

> ### ➡ Key points
>
> ◆ Once you have achieved consistency in your rest and activity, you could experiment with gradual increases in what you do physically and mentally
>
> ◆ It is important not to be too ambitious to start with
>
> ◆ This approach has been proved to help many people with CFS/ME

There are two stages in achieving an increase in what you can do. The first is to stabilize your current level of activity and to look at all the other ways in which you can help your body, such as relaxation, better sleep, good diet, and pain management. Once you have put into practice some of the things we have talked about in the previous chapters and have adjusted to a level of physical and mental activity that you can manage each day, you can move onto the next stage. This is to start increasing your activities **gradually**.

You may decide that you would get a better quality of life if you concentrated on increased physical activity. In Chapter 14 we discussed the kinds of exercise that are helpful for someone with CFS/ME. You could start with just a small amount of some of these (perhaps only 5 minutes to begin with) and then go on to increase the time by a minute or two in gentle stages. This is the sort of approach that is used in the graded exercise therapy (GET) that we discuss in Chapter 32.

However, you may find it more helpful to think about increasing your general activity, looking at **all** the things you do—physical, social, and mental—and increasing them slowly and carefully.

When you first start this increase, it is very important not to be overambitious. For instance, if you are at present comfortable doing one particular thing for 10 minutes, you could try the experiment of increasing it to 11 or 12 minutes (instead of doubling it as some people do). Another way would be to do it for 6 minutes, but then repeat it later in the day.

You may perhaps feel that by suggesting this sort of thing we are implying that you have been lazy and not trying hard enough. We certainly are not suggesting anything of the sort. Up till now you have probably been trying very hard, perhaps even too hard, and have been as active as seemed possible, but perhaps in the wrong sort of way.

## Reluctance to try increasing activity

You may be tempted to say 'I've tried this sort of thing before and it didn't work. It made me much worse'. There may be a reason for that. Perhaps you were too ambitious or had not managed to stabilize your activity at a sustainable level before you tried increasing it. We suggest that you try this experiment again—but do it carefully and follow the suggestions above.

If you were previously very active, the increase in activity you are planning now may seem too small to be useful—you might even think that it is pathetic. Tell yourself that every journey begins with a single step Compare your achievements with what you have been able to do since you have been ill, not with what you could do before!

If you have a very severe form of the illness, you may find it hard to believe that any increase in activity could be possible for you. We assure you that we know patients who were almost totally bedridden who have improved their condition by trying this kind of approach. In such cases it may be necessary to start with something very small, perhaps something as restrained as sitting up in bed for 5 minutes once a day and then increasing it to 6 minutes. That would be an important start that you could build on.

## Setting targets

It is worth thinking about definite targets. Instead of thinking 'I'd like to be able to walk much further', try a much more specific target such as 'I'd like to be able to walk to the park and back'. Then think about building up to that distance in stages over several weeks, or longer if necessary. Similarly, you can set a target for mental activity and again build up to that in stages. You may find it helpful to give yourself a period of total relaxation immediately after each activity. Activities that involve both physical and mental exertion are likely to be doubly tiring, so be cautious about those at the beginning. Do remember to build in pleasures as well as chores!

## What to expect when you start

Do not be alarmed if your symptoms increase a little. That is completely normal and to be expected. As long as the increase is minor and does not last for more than a few days, you do not have to worry. You will not be doing yourself any harm. In fact, this is evidence that you are increasing your ability to cope with activity. You will adjust to this increased level of activity. Do not increase your activity for a week, and see if your symptoms ease off. Then stay at this level for a week or two before making another increase. If your increased symptoms persist, you may have made too big an increase. Slow down a little, wait for a bit, and then try again but with a smaller increase. Sometimes you may need to stay at a certain level for 2 or 3 weeks before moving on again. If you feel very ill, you may have to ease off for a while and then start increasing again when you feel a bit better.

However, there are various pitfalls along the way. If you know what to expect, it will be much less scary:

- You are likely to feel a bit worse when you start this sort of programme. You are not doing yourself permanent damage if you get a mild increase in symptoms. You just need to adjust to a new level of activity. This sort of programme has been tried out in many CFS/ME clinics and has been proved to be safe and to work. Do not give up just because you feel a little worse, even though it may be very tempting to think that you should go back to resting more.

- At a time when you are about to start another increase, you again may feel a bit worse, but this is likely to be due to feeling a bit nervous about it.

- If things are working well, you may well be tempted to go ahead too fast, do too much, too soon, and crash. Taking things slowly without being too ambitious will be much more successful in the long term. Do your best to stay disciplined.

- Life can get in the way. You may have unexpected demands on your time and energy—a minor crisis, an unplanned visit, or a birthday. Just let it happen and then go back to your programme later.

- Improvement never happens in a straight line kind of way. You are bound to have times when you feel worse for no apparent reason. Do not be cast down by this or believe that it means the programme is not working. Stick with it and wait for things to improve again.

This kind of gradual increase in activity may take quite a time to achieve significant results. It depends very much on your illness and on how long you have been ill. Do not despair because it seems that improvement is not happening as quickly as you would like. If you keep going, there is a very good chance that you will achieve a very much better quality of life. This sort of approach to treatment has been validated by proper research trials as well as by clinical experience away from research.

## Getting someone to help you

It can be very helpful to have someone working with you while you do this kind of programme. You may be able to find a health professional experienced in this sort of thing who can supervise your progress, discuss the problems you encounter, and encourage you to persevere. If you cannot find someone like that, you may be able to involve a friend or a relative, though it should be someone you really trust. Reporting your progress can be a real incentive. However, it definitely is possible to do it on your own, though probably you will need to move at a slower pace than if you had back-up.

Once you have achieved a pattern of consistency in your life, you could try the experiment of making cautious and controlled increases in both physical and mental activity. Setting goals for such increases and working carefully towards them is helpful. This approach has been proved to help many patients.

# 20

# What gets in the way of being sensible?

## ➡ Key points

- Sticking to a pacing programme can be difficult. Things get in the way

- Identifying what stops you pacing yourself well is the first step in overcoming this problem

- Doing too little can sometimes be as much a problem as doing too much

- It is helpful to learn from times when you pace yourself successfully

You may decide that a pacing programme is a good idea, but it is very likely that you will find that sticking to it is not that easy. You will probably find things get in the way—some coming from outside pressures, but some coming from your own beliefs and emotions. Clinical experience and research both show that identifying the things that stop you pacing yourself as well as you could is extremely important in this kind of self-help programme. When you know what these barriers are, you can look for ways round them.

We can tell you of some of the most common things that get in the way of being sensible and suggest possible ways of getting round them, but you will need to recognize and identify which of them applies to you. It may help if you keep a diary for a while, recording what you are doing, what you are thinking, what is happening at the time, and what the results are. If you can catch your fleeting thoughts just **before** you start doing something or at the moment when you decide to go on doing it for longer, it is likely to give you far greater insight into what pushes you into overactivity. You may be surprised to find that some of your motives for doing or not doing things are not as reasonable as you thought.

# Doing too much

Most people are driven by imperatives—'oughts', 'musts', and 'shoulds'—often going back to childhood. If you think about yourself, you might be able to recognize some of your own. Typical ones can be 'If you have started something, you really ought to finish it', 'You must try to do better than that', 'You should be getting on with things instead of just sitting around doing nothing', or 'If you aren't nice to people they won't like you'. You might even be able to hear the adult voice saying that to the child you used to be and challenge that voice as not being appropriate today.

Typical thoughts that you can begin to recognize as danger signals could be ones such as 'I'll just finish it and then I'll rest', 'I know I'm tired, but I must get this finished', 'People will think I'm being a wet blanket or selfish if I don't join in their plans', 'I'm tired of being sensible' or 'I must look after my family in the way I used to'.

So here are just some of the things we have heard about from other sufferers. Thinking about these may give you some guidelines, but you will need to recognize the things that specifically get in **your** way.

## Pressures of just surviving

For a lot of people with CFS/ME—those living on their own, mothers with young children, people with unsupportive families, those struggling to keep on with a job—just doing the minimum to keep going can make overactivity almost unavoidable. It can help if you can stand back and look at all that you believe needs doing and consider whether **some** of it might not be absolutely essential. It might be possible to restructure the way in which the essential is done, breaking tasks down into smaller bites and stopping for a rest between each one.

## Lack of authoritative management advice

It is much easier to pace yourself and to 'sell' this idea to others if you can say 'I am pacing myself in this way because my doctor tells me it is essential' rather than just 'I have found from experience that this is the best way of managing my illness'.

Nevertheless, if what you do say is said with total confidence, it is much more likely to be received with belief and acceptance. Building up your confidence in your own judgement and expertise is vital.

## Other people's expectations

It is only too easy to get sucked into doing too much by what you believe other people are expecting from you. It is worth considering three things:

◆ Are your ideas about their expectations accurate? Could you check what they really do expect?

◆ Are their expectations of you unreasonable? Could you communicate with them better, so that their ideas are more realistic?

◆ How important is it to you to fulfil their expectations? Do you really need to please them if they are being unrealistic?

## Your own model of a 'good person'

We all have an internal model of what a 'good person' is and does. Trying to match up your activities with this model when you are unwell is more than likely to lead you into doing too much. Your model of yourself may have worked for you before you were ill (though it might have been one of the things that led you to overdoing it even then) but does it fit in with the way you are today? Could you change it for something more appropriate to your present circumstances, perhaps by thinking about your value from 'being' rather than from 'doing'?

> Sharon felt that she ought to be doing more for and with her children. She felt that she would be a bad mother if she looked after herself instead of concentrating on them. After a while though, she came to see that she was of value to them by just being there, able to listen to them when they needed to talk, and that if she pushed herself into complete exhaustion she was able to do less for them. Being 'good enough' was better than trying to be perfect!

## Being a perfectionist

This can be one of the things that really get in the way of being sensible. If you still believe that everything you do has to be done to a very high standard, you are likely to push yourself hard—probably far harder than is appropriate for the way you are now. You could try looking at the advantages and disadvantages of being a perfectionist. Why do you need to be so hard on yourself? What is wrong with being average? Are you imposing standards on yourself that you would not expect from someone else in your position?

If you find it hard to shift from being a perfectionist, you might try telling yourself that the pacing programme takes priority and concentrate on doing that in the very best way possible.

## Wanting more of a rare pleasure

If your life is restricted by illness, it is very tempting to prolong a 'rare pleasure' 'This is lovely; I want more of it **now**' and so move from allowable fatigue into sheer exhaustion. Try to remind yourself that by stopping in time there is a much better chance of having pleasure tomorrow, rather than feeling very unwell.

## Impatience

It can be very easy to slip into the trap of wanting to get something finished and out of the way, and so keep on doing it for too long. Again, try to remind yourself that stopping in time will give you a greater chance of achieving things later. You can always come back and finish it when you have had a rest.

## A desire to catch up on things after a bad spell

If you have had a time when your CFS/ME has been worse and then find yourself feeling a bit better, it is very easy to leap into overactivity in sheer relief. You may think of 'better' as a chance to catch up on all the things that have had to be left undone. Try to hang onto the belief that discipline is just as important in the good times. Actually, it is probably even more important.

## Pride

Many people find that pride gets in the way of good pacing. They resent asking for help or feel that they would be less of a person if they dropped their standards. You might consider the difference between self-respect and pride. Self-respect is important; pride is not.

## Getting carried away by an activity

When you are doing something absorbing, it can be very easy to go on too long and only notice rather too late just how tired you have become. Setting time limits for yourself is a good idea. Work out how long you can do a particular activity before getting too tired and try to stick to just that length of time. You could use a kitchen timer or an alarm clock to remind you when you have done enough. You can always come back to the activity later when you have had a rest.

# Doing too little

So far we have only mentioned the factors that can lead to doing too much, but doing too little can also sometimes not be sensible. It can be very helpful to think about what you avoid doing and why you avoid it. These are some of the reasons people with CFS/ME have told us.

## Fear

CFS/ME can be such a bewildering condition, particularly if you have not been given authoritative guidance about how to manage it, that it can be difficult to be certain how much you can safely do. Consequently, it can feel safer to avoid activity for fear of making yourself worse. We hope that this book will help you understand more about what is possible and safe.

If you did something and felt very ill afterwards, you will quite justifiably feel nervous about trying it again. However, it could be that you did too much of it or you did it at a time when you were already tired from doing something else. That activity might be within your capacity now if you timed it better or did it for a shorter time.

Most people with CFS/ME have one particular symptom that they dislike or fear more than the rest. They are likely to be very dubious about doing anything that seems to provoke that symptom. It is always worth remembering that none of the symptoms is in itself dangerous. It may help if you can change your thinking from 'This symptom is dangerous' to 'I don't like this symptom, but I don't have to fear it'.

## Wondering what other people will think

You may well be nervous that if other people see you doing something out of the house they will disbelieve your illness. You may feel that they will think something like 'If they can do **that**, they can't really be that ill'. You may need to be prepared to explain that this is a rare pleasure and that other people do not see the times when you need to rest.

## The effort of motivating yourself

There may well be things that you need to do or would like to do that would be possible, but the effort of getting organized to do them can seem to be too much bother. This can be particularly true if your mood is low. It is worth reminding yourself that doing them is likely to make you feel better—maybe not physically, though that is possible, but because it would give you a sense of achievement.

### Doing things in the same way as before you were ill

There are likely to be many things that could be possible for you to undertake if you could tackle them in a rather different way. Forward planning and lots of advance preparation might make something possible that you have written off as not for you now. We talk more about this in Chapter 27.

## Looking at what you are getting right

So far we have talked about the things that are likely to push you into not managing what you do as well as you could. Another approach to good management is to identify the times and the circumstances when you have got the balance between rest and activity right. Recognizing your successes and building on them can be very helpful.

> Pacing yourself—doing enough but not too much—is a central part of your strategy for improvement. It really can help to spend some time looking at all the things that get in the way of this. At each stage of your illness you may need to think and re-think about what gets in the way of being sensible.
>
> Equally, you could benefit from identifying the times when you pace yourself well, so that you can build on your successes.

# 21

# Improving your mood

> **Key points**
>
> - Anything that you can do to improve your mood will help you feel better
>
> - There are things you can do to cope better with mood changes
>
> - You may need to deal with old problems as well as new ones
>
> - Counselling can be useful, particularly if you define what you want from it

In the previous chapters, we discussed some things you can do to help yourself in a practical way. In these next chapters we will look at the way you feel emotionally, which can be just as important.

We are well aware that many people with CFS/ME have to cope in a climate of disbelief. Their own doctor, their family, or their friends may suggest that their illness is somehow their own fault—that it is just psychological and that they should snap out of it by trying harder. In extreme cases, they may even be told that they are not really ill—they only think they are. That can make it very difficult to admit to having emotional problems. Even if you do find it difficult to discuss such problems with most other people, it will certainly help if you can find someone safe to confide in. You can at least admit them to yourself.

Mind and body cannot be separated. Emotions and moods have a physical effect on the body, and what happens to the body has an effect on mood.

This is true of **any** illness, not just CFS/ME. Anything that you can do to improve your mood or to deal better with such emotions as loss, anger, frustration, and fear can be an important part of your programme to help yourself. Keeping worry, anxiety, and stress within reasonable limits will take some of the pressure off your body.

# Mood

Having an illness like CFS/ME can be a very depressing and frustrating experience. If you often feel in low spirits, that is hardly surprising. Changes in mood are one of the recognized symptoms of the illness. You may find that you cry much more easily or get irritated by small things that would not have bothered you before you got ill. Often getting too tired can push you into low spirits.

As with any long-term illness, you are likely to have times when you experience feelings of loss, anger, fear, or frustration. At times these feelings may seem overwhelming, but with practice they can be managed. Anything you can do to lift your spirits will be of value. It may help if you can find someone who feels able to listen when you need to talk about what is happening to you. It often works better if that person is someone like a counsellor or a friend with whom you are not emotionally involved—talking about these sorts of things to a partner or a close relative can often end up with both of you getting distressed.

## Loss

You may grieve for the person you used to be before you were ill and for all that that person could do then. You may feel a sense of loss for some of your hopes for the future. We have spoken to many people who mourn these losses just as strongly as they would the death of a partner or a close friend. Talking about it will probably help, particularly if you can find someone to talk with who understands about bereavement.

## Anger

Anger can be a very stressful and fatiguing emotion, though often an under-standable one. Many people with CFS/ME feel enormous anger at their doctors for not being able to help them more or for not seeming to take their illness seriously. They often get very upset by other people not understanding what is happening to them. They may feel resentment at the poor support they are getting from those close to them (sometimes quite justifiably). This is a stage of illness that most patients go through, but it is important to move on from it. You do not want to get stuck in angry resentment. Improving your communication skills will probably reduce some of the areas of friction. We talk more about that in Chapter 25.

### Fear and anxiety about the future

It is not surprising that you sometimes feel afraid of what is happening to you and what it might mean for your future. One thought to hang onto is that although CFS/ME can be extremely unpleasant and debilitating, it is **not** life threatening. We hope that if you try some of the techniques we have suggested earlier you will begin to feel a little better and so become more optimistic about the future. There is life after CFS/ME, even though it may be hard to believe that now. Allow yourself times when you think constructively about your fears, but do not dwell on them all the time.

### Frustration

Frustration is also a quite understandable emotion in your circumstances. There is so much you would like to do that seems impossible now. You may be able to find ways in which you can do just a little more of what you want, particularly if you can break it up into smaller 'bites'. We talk more about this in Chapter 27. The more you can work on finding ways round your problems, the better you will get at it and the less frustrated you will feel. In Chapter 20 we talked about perfectionism getting in the way of being sensible. If you can allow yourself to accept slightly lower standards, even if just for now, you are likely to feel less frustrated.

### Feeling depressed

Depression is one of those words that can mean very different things to different people. At one end of the scale it can be used to describe a feeling of low spirits or a temporary misery; at the other end it can describe a persistent mood of deep despair. Many people with CFS/ME experience periods of low mood and misery (often associated with being overtired after doing too much). Managing your activities in the way we described in earlier sections will make this happen less. It can also help if you can remind yourself that this is something that will pass when you have had a rest. What doctors refer to as 'clinical depression' is something much more serious, for which you do need help. We talk about this in much more detail in Chapter 22.

## Maintaining self-esteem

It is important that you work to preserve and improve your sense of self-esteem. Giving yourself proper credit for any achievement, no matter how small, will help. Setting yourself small, realistic targets and achieving them can also help.

It is very easy to concentrate on what is going wrong. Paying as much or more attention to what you are getting right can help redress the balance. Thinking well of yourself is important. If you only look at what you are getting wrong, you are likely to have a lower opinion of yourself than if you pay equal attention to what you are getting right. One way to identify what works for you might be to keep a journal for a few weeks in which you only record successful events and good times. Once you can see what they were and how you achieved them, you can plan to do more in the same way.

It can also help if you are able to take pride in your appearance (at least some of the time), perhaps with a becoming, though easily maintained hairstyle, using make-up or shaving regularly even if nobody else can see the results, or buying a new item of clothing (mail order can be useful) will all have a good effect on your morale.

## Old problems

Some of the problems that you had before you were ill can still be with you. You may even find that you have more time to notice them now you are ill. Old anger, old grief, difficulties with relationships, and so on can add to present distress. Sometimes just bringing them out into the open and talking about them to a friend or relative can help. You may decide that you would benefit from some professional help. This could be something to discuss with your doctor, who is likely to be able to point you in the right direction.

## Stress

Most people with CFS/ME find that stress makes them feel worse. Too much stress will hold back improvement, but it is not possible to avoid stress altogether. However, you can work both on reducing some of the excess stress in your life and on managing the necessary stress better. The techniques of problem solving that we discuss in Chapter 24 will be helpful. Relaxation and calm breathing (Chapter 13) will reduce the physical effects of stress on your body. Some of the stress in your life may be the result of poor communication between you and the people around you. We talk in Chapter 25 about how this could be improved.

You may need to look at what particular things cause you stress and to think a bit about why this is. Talking it over with someone you trust can often help you to identify what causes you most stress and then to find better ways of dealing with it.

# Worry

Becoming ill is bound to produce many problems, and problems lead to more worry—about how you are going to cope practically and financially, about how long your illness will continue, and whether you are going to get worse— to add to any worries you already had. Managing worry, not letting it get out of hand, should be an important part of your strategy.

## Limiting your worry

In Chapter 15 we talked about giving yourself a defined 'worry time'. What you need to avoid is thinking round and round your problems most of the time (which will be distressing, tiring, and inefficient). If you can restrict your thinking about problems to just one time each day, you are likely to be able to deal with them much more effectively. If a problem comes into your mind at another time, acknowledge it but tell yourself that you will think about it during your worry time. Some people find that it helps if they make a note of the problem, so that they can be confident they will remember it and consider it later.

## Keeping things in proportion

If you have many problems and worries, they can add up until they seem overwhelming. It is a common experience in illnesses of many kinds that people view problems in a different way from how they did when they were well. Any problem can seem more threatening. Talking things over with some-one else can often enable you to get worries into perspective. With each diffi-culty, could you stand back a little and say to yourself 'This is not a threat; it's just a problem. I'll deal with it now or later, but I won't go on thinking about it all the time'?

## Dealing with worry

If you decide to try the experiment of giving yourself a 'worry time', how can you use it most effectively? It certainly will help if you are very structured in your approach. The first step is to separate out your worries; be specific about what they are, and set out to deal with them one at a time. The techniques of problem solving that we talk about in Chapter 24 will be useful in deciding what you can do about whatever is worrying you. Accept that some problems cannot be solved immediately. If so, put that worry aside for the time being and concentrate on things that you can deal with now. Quite often you will find that a worry looked at calmly during the day seems much less important than when it filled your mind during the night. Try to keep a sense of proportion and check on the accuracy of your fears. Once you have given your worries an airing, move on to distracting yourself from them.

## Distraction

Finding ways of distracting yourself is important. This usually means doing something else or thinking about something else, so that you can stop thinking about the worry for a while and give yourself a period of respite. Experiment with different distractions (doing something you enjoy or thinking about something else absorbing that will blot out the worry) and find out what works best for you.

# Counselling

People with CFS/ME who have the problems with mood that we have described often hope that counselling will help them, but have a rather vague idea of how or why. As counselling is often either expensive, or only for a limited period if free, it is worth while thinking carefully about what you want from it before you start. A definite goal like 'I would like to deal better with such-and-such' will enable you to get the most value from the counselling sessions. If you can select one or two topics that distress you the most, you can work on these with the counsellor. If you get those resolved, you can always move on to something else.

Anything that you can do to improve your mood will have a positive effect on your well-being. Think about ways in which you could start managing your feelings of loss, frustration, anger, and fear. If old problems are still bothering you, this could be a time to get help with them. Getting better at dealing with worry and with stress will also help. Counselling can sometimes be useful, particularly if you can define what you want from it.

## 22

# Managing anxiety, panic, and depression

➜ **Key points**

♦ Anxiety, panic and depression cause physical symptoms and can be treated

♦ Self-help techniques can be especially helpful

♦ Antidepressants often help

♦ There are non-drug treatments as well

Some people with CFS/ME also suffer from anxiety, panic, or depression, and you are certainly not alone if you do experience this sort of thing. You may perhaps have had a tendency for this kind of problem before you got ill, or it may be a new and unwelcome burden. Anxiety and panic are very unpleasant to experience, and produce physical symptoms; anything you can do to control these emotional states will be of benefit to your general well-being. Feeling really anxious most of the time will certainly put added pressure on your body. Panic attacks can be exhausting, leaving you feeling really ill afterwards. Depression can also cause physical symptoms, make fatigue worse, and reduce your motivation, making managing your illness harder.

## Anxiety

Clinical anxiety is different from just feeling a bit worried a lot of the time. For some people it can mean a constant feeling of dread. The fear giving rise to the anxiety may not be obvious. It might involve uncertainty about the future; it might be a feeling that your life is out of your control. Bringing fears out into the open and then deciding what to do about them will give you more sense of control. You may find that when you have identified your fears that they are excessive or exaggerated.

## Physical symptoms

One of the added problems is that a state of anxiety can produce physical symptoms that are very similar to those of CFS/ME. This can then add another worry about whether your illness is getting worse, which in turn can increase your anxiety. Physical symptoms of anxiety can include:

Fatigue, palpitations, breathlessness, sweating, dry mouth, nausea, diarrhoea, twitching and shaking, dizziness, difficulty concentrating, muscle tension, and aches. Fast shallow breathing (hyperventilation) may add a feeling of breathlessness and light-headedness.

## What helps?

It will certainly help if you can find out whether an increase in symptoms is due to anxiety and whether when you are less anxious they subside. All the techniques of relaxation, calm breathing, and distraction that we talked about earlier will help reduce the symptoms of anxiety. Talking things over with someone you trust may also be a good idea. We give details in the reading list of books (Appendix 3) that will help you in anxiety management. Research has shown that self-help techniques can be very effective.

Sometimes, however, the level of anxiety is too great for self-help to be enough, and professional help may be necessary. Your doctor or therapist might suggest that you try one of the antidepressants that have been proved be effective in reducing anxiety. You will certainly be helping your body if you give this a try. We talk more about antidepressants later in this chapter. Tranquillizers (sometimes called anxiolytics) can sometimes be useful for very short-term anxiety, but are better avoided long term. You may also benefit from a form of cognitive behaviour therapy (CBT) specially tailored for dealing with anxiety. There is more about this in Chapter 32.

# Attacks of anxiety

Some people with CFS/ME get episodes of severe anxiety and associated physical symptoms. These are called panic attacks. These attacks may be so severe that some people experiencing them fear that they will collapse or even die. Such episodes can lead to a fear of leaving home or going out alone in case something bad happens. This is called agoraphobia and can be very disabling.

## What helps?

Obviously panic attacks and the associated physical symptoms will add to the problems of CFS/ME, so learning how to manage and control them is important. One technique that may seem to help in the short term but actually makes things worse in the longer term is avoidance—avoiding the places or the circumstances in which panic attacks are likely to occur. Avoidance will make you feel better in the short term, but will lead to an unnecessarily restricted life. It is better to use the techniques we have described to manage the feelings of panic. There are techniques that have been proved to work.

It is always easier to deal with panic as it is starting, rather than when it has built up into a full-blown attack. If you can recognize the early warning signs, you can start the techniques of relaxation and calm, slow breathing that will damp down the physical reactions. You can also identify and examine your fears and check whether they are accurate. Has what you fear ever happened? Are you really dying—again!

If you have frequent panic attacks, you should seek help from your doctor or from someone trained to deal with such things. Both psychological treatment and antidepressant drugs can cure panic. Help is available, so do ask for it.

# Depression

Feeling low in mood some of the time is a normal reaction to having an illness such as CFS/ME. Many patients find that their mood goes down when they get exhausted. Pacing can help this. Getting better at dealing with your problems will give you a greater sense of control of your life. However, if you find yourself feeling really low for much of the time, it is very important that you should get help. If you find yourself thinking seriously about suicide, you really do need help. At this stage it is not that important whether your depression is a reaction to the difficulties caused by your illness or whether you were depressed before you became ill. It just needs treating.

## What is depression?

The symptom that most people associate with clinical depression is feeling down or low in mood, but there are many other symptoms as well. In fact it is possible to suffer from depression without feeling depressed! The condition can show up as anxiety or extreme irritability. It can produce symptoms such as fatigue, pain, lack of energy or motivation, difficulty concentrating, reduced libido (sexual interest and drive), inability to enjoy things, and lack of interest in food leading to weight loss. You may be thinking of some of your symptoms as due to CFS/ME, when they are actually caused by depression. In fact it can be difficult to differentiate between CFS/ME and depression.

If you have depression, it does not mean that you are weak or pathetic. Depression is an illness associated with changes in the brain (an imbalance of neurotransmitters) that leads to it not working so well. It can be tempting to think 'I'm not the sort of person to get depressed', but do you really know who does get depressed? Anyone can get depressed, and many famous and high-achieving people do. Accept that it is an extra burden for you now, but one that happily can be treated. You may need to be tolerant of family and friends if they find it easier to deny your depression.

## Antidepressant drugs

Your doctor may suggest that you try taking an antidepressant drug. You might well have concerns about doing this, so let's look more closely at some of them:

◆ Some people simply dislike the idea of taking these drugs, feeling that they should be able to manage their problems themselves. This is an entirely understandable and laudable view. However, if you could get better by your own efforts, you would already have done so. Whilst antidepressants will not change your problems, they will make your brain work better so that you are more able to deal with them. You do not have to think in terms of drugs **or** helping yourself. You can do both.

◆ Other people may think that their condition is not depression and therefore an antidepressant is not an appropriate drug for them. As we have said earlier in Chapter 6, the term 'antidepressant' is a bit of a misnomer. These drugs can also help pain, anxiety, and sleep. Rather than worry about the name, it may be better to try something that might help.

◆ Many people think that antidepressant drugs may be addictive or cause long-term harm. Thankfully this is not true. Some of the newer drugs may cause some increase in symptoms if they are stopped suddenly, but these are not addictive drugs and you will not be able to sell them in your local night club! Nor is there any evidence that they do harm, even when taken for years.

## How to take an antidepressant drug

All drugs have some side effects, and antidepressants are no exception to this rule. Starting with a small dose and building up gradually will reduce the chance of such effects. This can be particularly important for patients with CFS/ME who may be particularly sensitive to the side effects of drugs. However, in order to treat depression, it is important to work up to a dose that is known to be effective (the full therapeutic does as recommended by your doctor). The danger of only trying the drug at a low dose is that if it doesn't help you could end up rejecting something as ineffective which might have been helpful if you had taken it at a higher dose.

One of the curious things about antidepressants is that they take a while to become effective. Although you may benefit almost immediately from the sedative effect, you are likely to notice side effects before you get the full benefit. Most of these drugs do not start to have beneficial effects on energy and mood for at least 2–4 weeks after starting taking them at the therapeutic dose. Be prepared for a period during which you experience side effects but not much benefit. Do persist. To give the drugs a fair trial you should take them for 6 weeks at a full dose. Clearly if the benefits do not outweigh the disadvantages at this stage, it is a good idea to talk to your doctor about stopping or changing the drug.

Though no major harm can come to you from stopping any of these drugs suddenly, it is generally wise to reduce the dose gradually. This will also minimize any withdrawal symptoms.

## How to choose an antidepressant

Antidepressant drugs require a prescription. Your doctor will therefore guide you in which drug to take. An experienced doctor or a psychiatrist can select the antidepressant that is the most suitable for you. Some of the drugs have a sedative effect, which can be helpful if you are having problems with sleep. Others are somewhat energizing, which can be helpful if you have problems in getting going in the morning or in motivating yourself to action. Some drugs have more effect on anxiety than others. There is no one antidepressant that works best for people with CFS/ME. It is very much a matter of 'horses for courses', and you may need to try more than one.

## The different types of antidepressant

There are four main types of antidepressants that are commonly used to treat depression, though other drugs are used as well:

## The tricyclics

The advantage of these is that they have been used by millions of patients for over 40 years, so a lot is known about them. They are known to be effective and we can be reasonably confident that they have no long-term harmful effects. The disadvantages are that they are know to cause side effects—the principal ones being a dry mouth, reduction in the ability of the eye to cope with bright lights at night, and sometimes a tremor. Other side effects will be listed with the medicine. Many of these drugs are sedative, so taken at night they can aid sleep. Although the side effects sound unpleasant, many people prefer to stick to these tried and tested drugs. Examples can be amitriptyline (Tryptizol or Elavil), imipramine (Tofranil), and clomipramine (Anafranil). There are newer modifications of these such as dosulepin (Prothiaden; not available in the USA), lofepramine (Gamanil; not available in the USA), and trazodone (Molipaxin or Desyrel).

## The monoamine oxidase inhibitors (MAOIs)

The MAOIs are another older type of drug that are now enjoying something of a revival. These drugs are potentially of interest for the treatment of CFS as they seem to be particularly helpful for people afflicted by low energy and especially with a feeling of heaviness, 'leaden limbs', and increased sleep. The principal disadvantage of these drugs is that they work by affecting an enzyme in the body that occurs not only in the brain but also in the digestive system. This leads to people using these drugs being intolerant of a small range of food. The 'banned' foods are those that include a chemical called tyramine and include certain red wines (especially Chianti), wild game, yeast extract, and some cheeses. Eating these foods can cause some quite severe reactions. As long as these foods are avoided, a normal diet is possible. The older MAOIs include phenelzine (Nardil) and tranylcypromine (Parnate). A more recent version is moclobemide (Manerix; not available in the USA). This has less stringent dietary requirements, but many clinicians feel that it is not as effective as the older versions.

## The selective serotonin reuptake inhibitors (SSRIs)

The SSRIs raise the level of the chemical serotonin (one of the neurotransmitters in the brain). They are as effective as the older drugs, but are safer in overdose and have fewer side effects. However, they may not be as effective in reducing pain. The principal side effect is nausea. Common examples are fluoxetine (Prozac), sertraline (Lustral or Zoloft), citalopram (Cipramil or Celexa), and fluvoxamine (Faverin or Fluvox).

### The newer agents

Pharmaceutical companies are continually striving to develop more effective drugs that work rapidly and have fewer side effects. The advantage of these is that they represent the pinnacle of pharmaceutical development, but the disadvantage is that they have not been around for us to be certain that there are no long-term effects. Examples of these drugs include venlafaxine (Efexor) and mirtazapine (Zispin or Remeron).

## Multiple drugs

Doctors will sometimes give drugs in combination to people who do not respond to taking only one. This can sometimes be hazardous and so is usually only done on the advice of specialists. One such combination is a non-sedative drug in the morning and a sedative one at night. For example, many patients benefit from an SSRI such as sertraline taken in the morning and a sedative antidepressant drug such as trazodone taken at night. Such combinations should only be used under the supervision of a doctor.

## Non-pharmaceutical antidepressants

People who dislike taking the products of the pharmaceutical industry for whatever reason sometimes ask if it is appropriate to take herbal preparations that are claimed to have an antidepressant action. One such preparation is St John's Wort (*Hypericum perforatum*). There is some evidence that this herb has an action similar to the antidepressants described above. Some people do experience side effects from it, and like any drug it can conflict with other prescribed drugs, so you should always check with your doctor before taking it. In contrast to manufactured drugs, this apparently 'natural' alternative has the disadvantage that it is harder to be sure about the quality and the quantity of what you are taking. Whatever one thinks about the pharmaceutical companies, they produce drugs of great purity in very carefully controlled doses. It is very much harder to do this with herbal preparations.

# Non-drug alternatives

Some people with CFS/ME simply do not wish to take a drug or find that they are unable to tolerate the side effects of antidepressants, even if they start them off very slowly. This does **not** mean that there is nothing that can be done to treat depression. There are other ways of tackling the problem. CBT (cognitive behaviour therapy) was first developed as a treatment for depression, though it is now used for many other illnesses too. CBT for depression aims to help you be aware of the thinking that keeps depression going—thoughts that are 'pushing mood down'—and to work at changing them. It is a collaborative process between a patient and a therapist. We talk more about CBT in Chapter 32. Many research trials have shown that CBT can be as effective a treatment as antidepressants. Though it is very much easier to do CBT with the help of a trained therapist, it is possible to do CBT by yourself. We recommend self-help CBT books in the reading list in Appendix 3.

Other things can help too. One of the things that can trigger depression is to find yourself in a very difficult, distressing situation, over which you feel you have no control (which sounds very much like a description of CFS/ME if you do not know how to manage it). As you get better at actively managing your illness, you will get an increased sense that you are in control and that optimism about the future is possible. Research has shown that one way of doing this, called problem solving (see Chapter 24), can help with depression. Finding someone who will listen to you is always helpful, particularly if they understand about depression. It is important that you remember that this black patch will pass and that you will come out the other side.

Anything you can do to improve your mood and to cope better with anxiety, panic, and depression will be of real benefit to your health as well as making your life easier. You could read some of the self-help books we recommend, and practise the techniques they suggest. Depression is something that can and should be treated. It is not a sign of weakness. You do not need to feel ashamed of depression or hesitate in asking for help. There are treatments that work.

# 23

# Managing your thinking

**➔ Key points**

♦ Unhelpful and inaccurate thinking can make your life more difficult than it need be

♦ Recognizing and changing such thinking can be very helpful

Understanding the way you think—the way you view yourself, your life, and the world around you and your illness—can make a great difference to the way you cope. We all of us, well or ill, have established patterns of thinking. Some of these are helpful and some unhelpful, and they influence our feelings and our mood. Moods and emotions have a huge effect on how you feel generally, which is why we believe that actively managing your thinking is so important. Some of your beliefs and thought patterns may well have been appropriate in the past but no longer fit the person you are today.

We can point out some specific ways of thinking that are common in a lot of people and mention how they can get in the way of good management of CFS/ME, but you are going to be the best person to judge just how much any of them apply to you. We are **not** saying that the only reason you are still ill is because of the way you think. What we **are** saying is that changing some unhelpful thought patterns may make life better for you and make it easier for you to stick to your self-help programme.

## Unhelpful thinking

### Thinking that the worst is likely to happen

You may have got into the habit of always expecting the worst, of believing that if anything can go wrong for you it will. This can make things a lot more difficult if you have CFS/ME. You are likely to fear that any new symptom means that your illness is deteriorating or even that it is a sign of a life-threatening condition. If you expect things to turn out badly, you are likely to be hesitant at trying anything new.

## Black-and-white thinking

In this style of thinking, everything is either good or bad, helpful or unhelpful, perfect or a disaster. If you stick to just black or white, you can miss out on the interesting shades of grey in between. You are likely to consider that you are either perfectly well or hopelessly ill, when the realistic viewpoint might be that you are considerably improved, but not yet in good health. Things are either catastrophes or successes instead of a mixed bag of a bit of failure and a bit of success. You are likely to believe that if you do not do something perfectly you have failed, instead of thinking (probably more accurately) that you did pretty well in the circumstances.

## Negative thinking

This is very common, particularly if you are feeling a bit depressed. You are likely always to believe the worst, particularly about yourself and the way people are reacting to you. Typical thoughts could be:

◆ 'I'm a failure.'

◆ 'I always get things wrong.'

◆ 'Everybody dislikes me.'

◆ 'I'm never going to get better.'

If you look again at those last three thoughts, you will notice that they contain very absolutist words such as 'always', 'everybody', and 'never'. This is very typical of negative thinking, when other words such as 'sometimes' and 'some people' would be much more accurate, and 'never' could be replaced by a concept such as 'it may take a long time'. Identifying and challenging these negative thoughts and looking at alternative, more accurate ones can make things seem much better.

## Mind reading

This is a very common problem. You presume that you know what people are thinking about you and it is usually rather negative. 'They think I'm not trying hard enough'. 'They don't believe that I really am ill'. That **might** be true, but it probably is not. Check up on the accuracy of your beliefs, if necessary by asking others; this will give you a more accurate view.

## Believing that if a thing happened once, it will happen again

This covers things such as believing that if you failed once, it means that you will always go on failing. It can be important to challenge this, particularly when it comes to managing your illness and pacing. A typical thought would be 'I tried pacing myself last week and it didn't work. There is no point trying again'.

## The 'socially acceptable' model

Another important area to consider is your own model of what makes you a 'good person'. In a society that is very much concerned with achievement, you may well feel devalued by being able to do much less. If you have had to give up your job, your own sense of worth may also have sunk. The 'model' you had before you were ill may have suited you then (though it might have been one of the things that made you more vulnerable to CFS/ME) but it may be totally inappropriate to your state now. It can be very helpful to look at your own ideas and judge whether they are helpful or unhelpful. The 'good person' model can often lead to you believing that you ought to be doing more than is appropriate or worrying that you are not doing enough. Our impression is that women tend to be more susceptible to pressures in this way, often believing that they ought to give their own needs a lower priority than those of their families or of those around them.

## Guilt

Another thing that comes up a lot in chronic illness (not just in CFS/ME) is guilt. So many of the people we talk with feel guilty about some aspect of their illness. This is often tied up with the concept of 'blame'. You may find it helpful to consider whether you would blame someone else in your position for being ill. It can sometimes be very difficult to convince people with CFS/ME that when we suggest ways in which they could manage their illness better we are not blaming them for being ill, which we certainly do not. Some people tend to assume that if you become ill and stay ill it is somehow your fault. For people suffering from CFS/ME this may be made worse by the suggestion that they are really just lazy. These comments are ignorant and unfair, and can make managing illness so much more difficult. Don't assume that they are being made unless you are sure; if they are, ignore them.

# Challenging unhelpful thinking

So, what if you have decided that some of your thought patterns are unhelpful? What can you do about it? There are some well tried and tested methods of challenging faulty thinking. Mostly they consist of asking yourself questions such as the following:

◆ 'What is the evidence that supports this belief?'

◆ 'Would I apply these standards to somebody else I cared about?'

Once you recognize your unhelpful thinking you can challenge it—along the lines of:

◆ 'OK, that is one way of thinking, that is one interpretation of events. Are there any others?'

◆ 'What could I do to gather evidence to judge whether this thought is accurate?'

We talk about this in more detail in Chapter 32 and we give details in the reading list (Appendix 3) of some books that you could find helpful.

# Other things to consider

There are some other ways of thinking about yourself and your illness that can help or hinder your improvement.

## Aiming for normality

However severe your condition, there is more to your life than your illness. You are still a person of worth, even though you are ill, and you can contribute to life and take an interest in things other than illness. You do not have to think of yourself as **only** a person with CFS/ME. The more you concentrate on your illness and the difficulties of your life now, the worse you are likely to feel. 'Symptom scanning' is likely to make you notice symptoms much more and mind about them much more. Thinking and behaving in as normal a way as possible in the circumstances is going to make your life better. You need to balance pacing and sensible behaviour with the need to be 'ordinary'.

## Balancing acceptance and hope

So many people with CFS/ME who have got better tell us that they can look back and see that real improvement started when they **accepted** what was happening to them. 'This is not what I wanted. I do not have to like it, but it is what is happening today. How can I make the most of my material?'. This kind of acceptance does not mean that you have to give up hope for future improvement, rather the reverse. It is only when you are accurate in your thinking about today that you can start working on an improved tomorrow and so be more optimistic about the future.

Unhelpful and inaccurate thinking can make your life much more difficult than it needs be and can get in the way of managing your illness. Recognizing and challenging your unhelpful or inaccurate thoughts and beliefs is a useful tool to help you work on getting better.

# 24

# Dealing with problems

**➜ Key points**

◆ There are way of learning how to get better at dealing with problems and worries that will make you feel more in control of your life

◆ 'Problem solving' is one well-researched way of tackling problems

◆ You must choose one problem to work on at a time; some may be more easily solved than others

We all face difficulties and problems in our lives, and being ill can create a new batch to go with the ones you had before. At every stage of your illness things change; some problems get easier, but new ones crop up—even getting better can cause some problems! Managing problems in the best way is very much part of managing your illness and giving yourself the best chance of improvement.

Before going on to consider how best to deal with problems, you might like to think about the difference between difficult circumstances and problems. Many of the people we talk to seem to be trying to solve the difficult circumstances, rather than dealing with the problems that those circumstances produce.

As we said earlier, when you are feeling ill and tired, problems seem to loom larger. It is very likely that you will have times when **any** problem can seem very threatening. If you have lots of them, it can seem almost impossible to know where to start and how to find any solutions. Nevertheless, if you can hang onto the idea that they are just problems, not threats, you can do more about finding solutions. With each problem that you solve you will get better at dealing with others and you will build up confidence in your own abilities.

# Problem solving

One of the life skills that will be particularly useful to you now is called 'problem solving'. What follows is just a summary of the technique; in the reading list at the end of the book (Appendix 3) we point you to books you can read that will give you more guidance. What we suggest is that you start with just **one** fairly simple problem. You can then tackle it in seven stages.

## Stage 1: identifying and clarifying the problem

It is going to be much easier to tackle any problem if you can identify exactly what it is and separate it out from all the rest of the stuff that is bothering you.

◆ What exactly is the problem?

◆ When and where does the problem occur?

◆ What other people does it involve?

Be very specific; do not muddle it up with others. Give it a name. Write down a clear description of the problem.

> John had been ill for 3 years and was not well enough to work. He lived on his own, though he had a brother living nearby. He knew that he was letting his paperwork get out of hand. There were bills, official forms, and letters strewn around in a complete muddle, so that he spent a lot of time looking for a specific bit of paper and was often late paying bills. This worried him, but the whole thing seemed such a mess that he kept putting off dealing with it. He decided the problem was 'having paperwork not done'.

## Stage 2: deciding on your goal or goals

Set yourself a goal of what would change things for the better, rather than a somewhat vague hope for improvement. Choose a goal that you know you can achieve and make it very definite.

> John realized that he had two goals associated with this problem, to get his paperwork into order and to clear up the backlog of unanswered mail. He decided to tackle the sorting out first.

## Stage 3: thinking of as many solutions as possible

'Brainstorming' can be a useful technique. It is a good idea to use a pencil and paper at this stage. Your aim is to identify as many solutions as possible, writing each one down, and not stopping to think about whether any of them would work until you have run out of ideas. Having someone you trust doing this with you can be useful as they may be able to suggest ideas you might not have thought about. You do not need to reject **any** idea at this stage, even if it seems to be ridiculous. Do not stop and say 'Oh, but that wouldn't work'. Only when you have got your complete list in front of you should you start to evaluate them. Ask yourself what are the pros and cons of each solution.

John asked his brother to help him with the brainstorming. Together they made up a list of solutions that included paying someone else to sort things out, letting his brother do it for him, doing all of it himself right away, doing it himself but in smaller bites, and buying some coloured folders to file papers in.

## Stage 4: choosing the best solution and deciding how to put it into practice

When you have got your list of solutions in front of you and have thought about each one, you can choose the best solution. That is the one that seems to be the most practical and which fits your situation best.

John decided that he would prefer to do the sorting out himself, but not all at once which would be too tiring. He decided to set aside 20 minutes each day to sort papers. He would get his brother to buy him some coloured folders to put them in when they were sorted.

When you feel happy about the solution, break it down into steps. 'I could begin by doing this and then move on to doing that'. Be very definite about what you are going to do and when you are going to do it.

John decided that his steps would be:

♦ to go round gathering up all the papers and to put them on the dining table

♦ to sort them all out into piles—bills, official forms, letters to be answered, urgent items, etc.

♦ to label the folders

♦ to put each group of papers into the appropriate folder in date order.

He would make sure that he did at least 20 minutes every day, though if he felt up to it he would come back to the task later in the day.

## Stage 5: trying it out

There is no point in having worked out a potential solution if you do not use it. If you start finding good reasons **not** to try out the solution, it probably was not the right one, or you may have chosen too big a problem to begin with and would perhaps do better to tackle just part of the problem.

Once John got going, he found that it only took him a week to get everything sorted. Having got things in order, he could see what needed doing urgently and what could wait.

## Stage 6: evaluating the success of the solution

When you have put the solution into practice, check on whether it is working. It can be helpful to discuss this with someone. You will have learned a lot from any mistakes you have made.

Though John had got things sorted out, it would still take him some time to catch up on the backlog of things he had not done, which worried him a little. He thought that it might have been better to have accepted some help from his brother. However, he felt that he could now start to work out a system that would keep things in order.

## Stage 7: beginning again

If the problem is solved, congratulate yourself. If not, start again at step one and decide if was the best problem to tackle. If you still think it was, try an alternative solution and progress through the stages as last time. You can then go on to tackle other problems in the same way.

Do keep in mind that some problems do not have obvious solutions or cannot be tackled yet because you do not have enough information. Part of your technique for dealing with problems should be to accept that some things may have to be tolerated for the time being. Another important part may be to accept that you may have to postpone doing any work on some problems until you have gathered more information. You cannot make realistic decisions without enough data.

Life is full of difficulties and problems, but getting better at dealing with them in a structured way will reduce stress and make you feel more in control of your life

- Identify the problem.

- Decide on your goal.

- Think of as many solutions as possible.

- Choose the best solution and decide how to put it into practice.

- Try it out.

- Evaluate its success.

- If that solution did not work, go back and try another solution. If it did work, move on to another problem.

- Accept that some problems cannot be solved just now.

# 25

# Better communication

➡️ **Key points**

◆ Clear, calm communication is most effective

◆ Learn techniques of better communication and practise them to get what you want with minimum effort

One of the things that can add to the difficulty of managing any long-term illness is poor communication between you and the people around you—family, friends, doctors, officials, employers, etc. Getting a message across clearly and calmly can do a lot to make a difficult situation easier and reduce stress, so it should definitely be part of your plan for helping yourself. Good communication is a skill that can be improved with practice.

These are some topics which we think are particularly relevant to your present situation.

## Quiet assertiveness

You will communicate better if you can be quietly assertive, but that is easier to do if you believe that you still have rights. It is all too easy to slip into the trap of believing that you have stopped having rights since becoming ill. It can be helpful to think about your own rights, taking your illness into account. You could try thinking about the rights you would give to somebody else in your circumstances such as:

◆ The right to look after themselves and not be pushed into doing something that would tire them too much.

◆ The right to say 'no'.

◆ The right to choose what help they accept.

◆ The right to use some of their energy for pleasure.

Balance your rights against the rights of the people around you. It is a two-way process. Other people have rights that need to be thought about.

Once you have a list of your own rights that feels comfortable to you, you will be in a much better position to be quietly assertive about what you want and what you need.

## Explaining an invisible illness

It is very natural that you should want the people around you to understand what is happening to you, and their lack of understanding can be a cause of friction and distress. CFS/ME can be an invisible illness. Fatigue, malaise, and pain may not show. Often people only see you when you are well enough to get out or to see visitors, so they tend to judge you by how you appear then. Though more people are learning about CFS/ME, there is no reason why they **ought** to understand unless they are given the facts. (Did you know much about it before you became ill?) It is always worth checking up on what other people do or do not know and then filling in the gaps. Do not expect them to understand what you have not told them. You have a right to choose whether or not to tell some people about your CFS/ME, but you have to accept that if you do not tell them they may think of you as a well person.

Sufferers often want **all** the people around them to understand **all** about the illness, but it can be worth thinking about this in a more specific way. Try thinking about one particular person. What do you feel that you are not getting from that person because of their lack of understanding? Then ask yourself these questions:

◆ What particular aspect of your illness do you want them to understand?

◆ What information would help them understand?

◆ What would they say or do to show that they did understand?

◆ Is what you want something they can give?

◆ Is it reasonable to expect them to give it to you?

Once you have got that clear in your mind, you can start thinking about what information to give them and how to explain your reasonable needs. It may take time for them to adjust to this approach.

### Asking for help

Many people find it difficult to ask for help. Some feel that they **ought** to be able to cope on their own and that it is a sign of weakness if they do not. Some fear rejection 'What if they said no!!'. It is worth looking at your own feelings about this. A good working motto is 'I can ask anyone for anything as long as I respect their right to say no'.

### Saying 'no' yourself

You may find it very hard to refuse when you are asked to do something for or with someone else (though it should be on your 'rights' list to refuse if it would be too tiring or interfere with your pacing programme). One approach that can sometimes help is to turn down the whole request with a show of regret, but to offer something much smaller instead, e.g. 'I can't come away for the weekend but I'd love to come to tea'.

## Practical suggestions

These are some suggestions for better communication that have been proved to help:

♦ Try to stay calm. There is something about strong emotion that makes people discount much of what you say. This is particularly true when talking to young people; emotion in a parent seems to produce selective deafness in teenagers! Anger certainly gets in the way of getting your message across.

♦ Keep it short and simple. Long-winded explanations often make people lose interest.

♦ If possible, tap into the experience of the people you are talking to. For instance, if you are trying to explain the overwhelming exhaustion you may experience, try reminding them of a time when they experienced something similar (like reminding a mother what it was like when she had a teething baby keeping her awake at night as well as an active toddler). When you have pointed out what is similar, you can outline the differences—that is, it may not take much to get you exhausted and a 'good night's sleep' probably will not make you feel much better.

- Try to stand back sometimes and look at things from the other person's point of view. If you feel that you have good cause to complain about what they are doing (or not doing), try to stick to criticisms of their actions, not of them as people.

- Do your best to stay consistent, even though your condition may fluctuate. Try not to turn down help crossly one day when you are feeling a bit better and then be wounded another time because help is not offered.

- If someone asks you how you are, it is better not to answer 'Fine' automatically. If you usually say you are fine, people will assume that that is how you are. On the other hand, saying too much about how terrible you are feeling can make some people switch off. Try to find a balance between the two approaches.

- Give them something to read. This book might be a start!

If you have a specific point you want to get across, you will probably do better to write down in advance what you need to say, particularly if you have problems with memory and concentration. This can be a great help when you are talking to doctors or officials. You can then be sure that you have covered all the necessary points. Show that you appreciate that their time may be limited and keep it as brief as you can without missing out on anything important.

> Clear, calm communication will reduce stress and save energy. If that is something you find difficult, read about it and practise your skills. The more you work at it, the easier it will become.

# 26

# Managing relationships and people

**➔ Key points**

♦ Working on improving relationships may be difficult but it is usually worthwhile

♦ Relationship are a two-way processes, so remember to think about the other person's point of view as well as your own

♦ The relationship you have with your doctor is an important one and worth working on

Being ill often changes relationships. Even the best relationships can be put under strain, and one that was a little rocky to begin with may become very difficult. You may be grieving for the past, for your lost job perhaps or the things that you cannot do now. However, people close to you may also have lost by your illness. A carer may have had to have taken on the responsibility of housework or earning the money, and have had to give up a lot of things they previously enjoyed on their own or with you. Their grief needs to be acknowledged too. You may feel that they are not caring enough; they may feel that you are asking too much. There may be resentment on both sides.

A difficult relationship is an obvious cause of stress, which will not be helpful to you in your plan for improvement, so anything you can do to ease the relationship will be of benefit. There are no absolute rules; each person and each relationship is unique but some general guidelines might be:

♦ Keep communications open. Avoid 'mind reading' (that is, assuming that you know what the other person is thinking in a given situation). You could well be inaccurate in your assumptions.

◆ Check that the other person in the relationship knows the facts about your illness. Find simple ways of explaining how it affects you.

◆ If something in the relationship is bothering you, choose a time when you are both at your best to discuss the problem. Some people find that it helps to have a definite time once a week to talk over problems, with both sides having equal time to put their side of the picture without being interrupted. Spend a little time imagining yourself in their place and thinking about things from their point of view. This can often let you see that they are not being totally unreasonable.

◆ Accept that some people are not going to understand what your illness is like for you. With some friends or relations you may have to choose between continuing to seeing them in spite of their lack of understanding or cutting out that relationship for the time being. Some people do feel very uneasy about illness (it reminds them of their own potential vulnerability).

◆ In general, try to aim for negotiation rather than confrontation.

> Bertha was very distressed and angry that her family were still expecting her to do all the housework in spite of her illness. After a while she realized that just moaning at them was not getting her anywhere. Instead, she chose a time when all of them were at their best and set up a family conference. She itemized all the things that needed doing and explained why she really was not capable of doing them all. She asked them to make suggestions as to which tasks each individual would prefer to do (rather than giving them orders) and then negotiated towards a solution that they all felt was fair.

◆ If relationships get very difficult and strained, it may be helpful to seek professional help—family therapy or couple therapy for instance. Your doctor will probably be able to make suggestions as to how you could find this help.

## Sexual relationships

If you have a partner, one of the areas that can cause difficulties and stress is that of your sexual relationship. If you are very tired or in pain, sex can be the last thing on your mind. Nevertheless, it is an important factor in your relationship. You may need to educate your partner so that he or she can consider positions and methods that are easier for the one with CFS/ME and also to think about different timing. Would mornings or afternoons be a better time for you than last thing at night? Do believe that sex does not necessarily have to be just about passion; warmth and affection, closeness, and cuddling can be just as important. Sex can be energizing as well as exhausting.

## Improving your relationship with your doctor

If you have an illness that is not going to improve quickly, having a good relationship with your doctor can make a great deal of difference. Even if it is not very good at the moment, it may be possible to improve it.

Sometimes people with CFS/ME expect too much from their doctors. It can be helpful to distinguish between what you **need** from doctors and what you **want** from them—you **need** appropriate medical treatment (which is what they were trained to do); you may **want** a degree of emotional support (which they may feel is not their role).

Once you are clear in your mind about what you need from your doctor, it can be very helpful to look at things from his or her point of view. Doctors these days have been trained to make diagnostic tests and then apply a treatment based on the results of those tests, so a condition like CFS/ME can be difficult for them.

These are suggestions about getting on better with doctors, based on what they have told us and what people with CFS/ME have told us:

◆ Doctors are often unhappy about the names ME or CFIDS for the condition as they feel they are technically inaccurate. It is probably more tactful to use the term CFS when talking to them (whatever you may call it to yourself).

◆ Doctors often dislike patients doing too much self-diagnosis (after all, it is what **they** were trained to do). It is generally better not to say 'I am sure I have got ME', but rather to describe your symptoms and then say something more indirect such as 'It has been suggested that I might have something like CFS'.

◆ Try to understand things from the doctor's point of view. Doctors like to make people feel better. CFS/ME can be frustrating for them too. They work by looking for things that they **can** treat.

◆ Try not to be angry if your doctor suggests that you might be suffering from depression. The physical symptoms of depression and anxiety can be quite similar to those of CFS/ME. Your illness may have features of both

CFS/ME and depression. Doctors know that they can suggest treatment for depression.

◆ Show that you realize that your doctor's time is limited. Write down the points you want to cover and the questions you want to ask so that you can express yourself clearly and briefly. If you have a great deal to discuss, consider asking for a double appointment.

◆ Do not expect your doctor necessarily to feel the same about alternative therapies as you do. He or she may not be comfortable with treatments that are not scientifically proven to work.

◆ Many people with CFS/ME only see their doctor when they are well enough to get to the surgery or office. Keep your doctor informed about what it is like at the bad times.

◆ Being a patient with a chronic illness can be quite different from the days when you just visited a doctor for something specific such as a sore throat. You may be able to discuss this new relationship with your doctor and together work out a new 'contract'.

◆ If you cannot get to the doctor, or have trouble choosing the right words when you do, trying writing a brief letter explaining the problem and saying what you want.

Your relationship with your doctor is an important one, so anything you can do to improve the partnership between the two of you will be of real benefit.

> Working to improve relationships may be hard work, but it will be of benefit to you. Remember that any relationship is a two-way process, so try to consider their side as well as your own. Being clear in the way you communicate is very important.

# 27

# Getting the best from today

➡ **Key points**

◆ It is worth working to improve your life today

◆ Look at what you are doing and see if it could be done in a more energy-efficient way

◆ It is important to include activities that give you enjoyment

We hope that by trying out some of the strategies for self-help we have outlined in previous chapters your condition will start to improve (even if only very slowly) so that you can look forward to a better tomorrow.

But what about today? Improving the quality of your life today is something worth aiming for. You are bound to have times when you are frightened that you are never going to get any better and that what you are today is all you will ever be. It may be an exaggerated fear, but it can still be there. Making today better can reduce fears about tomorrow. These are some practical suggestions about how to improve today.

## Making the most of a limited energy budget

At this stage you may well have to accept that the amount you can do is limited, so it is worth thinking about whether everything you are doing is essential or pleasurable. Some people find it helpful to think in terms of a budget for their energy expenditure in the same way they would budget a low income. You may have to make choices about whether you can afford something, whether it is in energy or money.

You could also think about whether you are 'spending' your energy efficiently. Using the same amount of energy to achieve a bit more is often possible if you think about it in a rather structured way. A good place to start is by considering your activities, mental as well as physical, under the headings of what, why, how, and when.

◆ *What*—could you reduce some of the things you do now by concentrating on essentials?

◆ *Why*—could you look at the reasons why you are doing what you do? Could it be because you have always done such-and-such, even though that is not really appropriate for you today?

◆ *How*—could you do the essentials in a more labour saving way?

◆ *When*—could you spread your activities out during the day and during the week?

## Changing the way in which you do things

If you are still doing things in the same way as you did before you were ill, you are likely to hit against obstacles and deny yourself possible pleasures or satisfactions. You may need to change your style quite a bit. One of the techniques that will help is to do a lot of forward planning, spreading out the task and pacing yourself carefully. Being too much of a perfectionist will certainly get in the way.

Clare used to enjoy having friends round for a meal and had very high standards when she entertained. After a few bad experiences, trying to do things in the same old style, she realized that her friends did not expect her to do so much. She thought about very simple food that could be prepared well in advance—something like a casserole and a cold pudding—and got almost everything ready the previous day. To her delight she found that the social occasion was just as successful as before and yet it did not exhaust her.

With anything that you would like to do but which seems beyond you at the moment, think carefully about whether it would be possible if you spread out the preparations in the previous day or days and kept things simple.

## Equipment

You may decide that there are various pieces of equipment that would make your life easier or allow you to do more with your available energy. Before you invest in anything expensive though, it can be worth asking yourself whether it is something you would still use if you got a bit better. Obviously, something like a microwave oven or a deep freezer could be useful, whatever your state of health. However, it is better not to rush into getting 'invalid aids' unless you really need them.

There may be small or inexpensive things that would make your life easier—even a more efficient can-opener could be helpful.

## Building pleasure into your life today

If you are feeling tired and ill it can be hard to think about enjoying yourself. You may have a puritanical feeling that you do not deserve pleasure while you are ill or you may feel that people will criticize you for using some of your available energy on things other than the essentials. However, pleasure is an essential part of your diet—just as important as good food. Often the things that used to give you pleasure are not possible at present, but that does not mean that you could not enjoy yourself in rather different ways. Now could be the time to try something a bit different.

You could try making a list of all the things you can think of that might give you pleasure or satisfaction, within the limits of your present condition. Keep it by you and add to it every time a new idea occurs to you. You might be surprised by how long a list you end up with.

Most people have things that they have always wanted to do but never had the time to try. This could be your time to do just a few of them. This could also be a time for you to learn more about subjects that have always interested you. Education does not have to be just about vocational training; it can be satisfying in its own right. Many people with CFS/ME find that this is a time to explore their creative side—art, writing, etc.

You know yourself and what you might enjoy. Experiment, always remembering that fun is possible and that it will do you a lot of good. You really do have the right to enjoy yourself and indulge yourself.

## Treats and rewards

One way of looking at things could be to imagine what you would do for friends in similar circumstances. You might buy flowers for them, pick out an amusing book, choose a nice video, and get some food that you know they enjoy. Have you considered indulging yourself in this way? Why not give yourself these sorts of little treats, if only as a reward for the way you are coping with your illness?

# Keeping in contact with the outside world

Unfortunately, being ill can mean that you lose out on a lot of the social activity you enjoyed before. Feeling isolated can be a very common problem for people with CFS/ME. Social contact is a basic human need and very necessary for you now. You may like to think about being social in a different way, such as having a friend join you for a take-away meal instead of inviting several people round for a meal you prepared yourself.

You may also need to replace the friends who dropped away because they could not cope with you being ill. Making new social contacts can often seem difficult, but usually there are ways round the problem. There may be a CFS/ME support group in your area that you could join and meet people with similar problems, though these groups do vary enormously and you may find that your local one is not your style. If you cannot get out easily, there may be local organizations that do home visits (perhaps one of the churches near you).

Socializing does not have to happen face to face. Pen friends (a postcard even if you cannot manage a letter) and telephone contacts can be very helpful. A lot of people with CFS/ME find that telephone calls are a lot less tiring anyway. You could also try e-mail. Anything you can do to keep in contact with the world is going to be good for you.

Improving the quality of your life today is very important, both for making life easier and to reduce fear and frustration. It can help if you look at all aspects of your life and think hard about small ways of making things a little better.

## 28

# Managing employment

➡ **Key points**

If you are still managing to hold down a job or are planning to return to work you might want to use the following techniques:

♦ Pacing

♦ Stress management

♦ Good communication

♦ Problem solving

You may still be working (even with great difficulty) or you may not be working but have made enough improvement to be able to think about getting back to work. What would be the best way of managing employment without putting too much strain on yourself? As we have said before, each person and each situation is different, so there are no hard and fast rules. However, we can offer some general, tried and tested suggestions.

First of all, it can be a great help if your employer, your immediate superior, and your colleagues know about your illness and understand what it involves. Of course this is not always desirable or possible. In some situations, it may have an adverse affect on career prospects to have it known that you have a health problem; some employers may be reluctant to take on a new employee with a record of ill health. You will have to be the best judge of this but, if you can be open about it; it will certainly make things easier.

You may have to accept that for a while you will have to limit what you do in the evenings and at weekends, and concentrate your energies on the working day. Pacing while you are at work is very important. Try to give yourself pauses during which you switch off and relax.

Everything we have said earlier about stress and stress management is particularly relevant in a working environment. It is worth giving a good deal of thought as to how you could reduce stress. Maybe you could go for a less demanding job; maybe you could get better at saying 'no' when unreasonable demands are made of you.

Communication and negotiation skills will certainly make your life easier. If the people around you do not understand about the limitations imposed on you by your condition, they may be resentful that you do not seem to be 'pulling your weight'. This would add to your problems.

One of the books in our reading list will give you more ideas about how to manage your working life.

> If you are still managing to hold down a job or if you are planning to return to work, then pacing, stress management, good communications, and problem solving will all help.

# 29

# Thinking about the future

## ➔ Key points

- Getting better can be wonderful, but it can also pose challenges

- Voluntary or part-time work may be the best route back to full-time employment

- Relationships may have to be re-defined as you improve

- You need to plan in advance how you would deal with a relapse

You may feel so stuck in your present problems that it is hard to envisage a better future, but the possibility is certainly there. If your health improves, you would begin to see things opening up, some of which could seem pretty scary. If you have been ill for some time, getting back into the world, perhaps coming off benefits and going back to work, can seem very daunting. There are likely to be problems about being better just as there have been problems about being ill. The more you can be clear about what the problems might be and what you might be able to do about them, the less scary it will be.

## Getting back to work

When you reach the stage at which you can see the possibility of working again, you will need to think about whether you want to return to your old job. If you do, it will obviously be easier if you have kept in touch with your previous employer and can negotiate a gradual return—perhaps part-time to begin with or in a less demanding role.

You may now recognize that your previous occupation is no longer attractive to you. It could be that the stress involved in your previous job was one of the factors that made you vulnerable to illness. Your previous job may no longer be open to you. This could be a good time to review what you want to do in life. One technique that many people find helpful is to think hard about their previous job and analyse which bits were stressful, which bits were bearable (though perhaps boring), and which bits were really enjoyable. Once you have identified what aspects of your work gave you the most satisfaction, you may be able to see a new direction that would include more of that sort of thing.

It may be that you now feel that you really do not want to return to your previous career. At this stage, all you may be certain of is that you do not want to go back to what you used to do, but have no clear idea of what else might suit you. This could be a good time to consider a wide range of other possibilities, without committing yourself to anything. Your period of convalescence provides you with an opportunity to 'play' with ideas before committing yourself. As all you are doing is thinking about it, you do not need to limit your ideas. 'Do I fancy being an astronaut? Well perhaps not'. Maybe what would suit you is something similar to what you used to do; maybe you feel that you need a complete change of direction. Think hard about your strengths as well as your weaknesses. Gather as much information as possible to help you in your decision making. Your local library will have books about career choices. You may be able to get some kind of career guidance. You could talk to people who are already working in an area that interests you. You could certainly use the problem-solving techniques we talked about in Chapter 24 on this.

## Voluntary and part-time work

Quite often the way back into employment can be through some kind of voluntary work, even if it is only for an hour or two per week. Just getting back into the world and doing something can be of benefit, but it could be even better if it is in an area that interests you. In that way you could get a taste of that kind of thing.

Voluntary work has other benefits. Many people find that they have lost confidence while they have been ill. Working with other people, even if you are not getting paid for it, can be one way of rebuilding that confidence. It can also be helpful to be able to say to a prospective employer that you have been doing something like this.

You may well be able to do a part-time job for a while without losing out on any benefits. Part of your information gathering may need to be talking to the officials administering your benefit to find out just how many hours you would be allowed to do or how much you would be allowed to earn without affecting your benefit. Later on, when you feel able to work longer hours, you could also investigate government schemes to help people with disabilities get back to work. If you are at present receiving permanent health insurance income, you could find out from the insurance company whether they allow part-time working while still getting some benefit.

Both voluntary and part-time work can be routes back to normal living.

## Education

Part of your plan for dealing with improvement might include education for a new career. You could start this in a very modest way, perhaps by just getting one book about a possible new direction and reading it slowly. Later on you may decide on retraining, but again this can be done modestly—taking one class a week to begin with and then increasing it later on when you feel up to it.

## Managing a relapse

Even if you seem to be improving steadily, there are likely to be times when you slip back a bit. Maybe feeling better will tempt you into doing a little too much, too quickly; maybe you will pick up an infection; maybe you will meet with an unexpected stress. Whatever the cause for a relapse, it can feel extremely frightening. You may tend to think in catastrophic terms 'I'm going back to where I was. I'm never going to get better again'. Of course that is not true. You will have just had a setback and can deal with it. Your forward planning needs to include thinking about how you would deal with a relapse. If you can think of a relapse as just a minor setback that can be managed as you have managed before, it will be much less frightening.

## Managing change

We have talked about getting back to work, but there will probably be other areas in which you will have adapt to a changed role as someone well rather than someone ill. You may have to move back to taking responsibility for things that you handed over to others while you were ill. You will probably need to work slowly at re-building your confidence at doing things on your own. You may need to think in terms of rehabilitation—such as getting used to driving again, perhaps with someone with you to start with and then short trips on your own. Doing things gently and not rushing into complete independence will probably make it easier.

While you were ill you might have had very little chance of meeting new people and have lost confidence in your social skills. Getting back to it can be difficult. Some people find that it helps if they deliberately seek out opportunities to meet people in a non-stressful way.

> Martin decided that one way to get back to socializing again would be to join a local weekly photography class. He would be likely to meet people there with similar interests. He was very nervous the first week, but found that it got easier. He enjoyed the class and made a couple of friends.

It is a fact of life, though one that may come as something of an unpleasant surprise, that not everyone will necessarily welcome your re-emergence into normal living. Some of the people around you may have got used to you being ill and actually enjoyed having you dependent on them. Because they found a role for themselves in being carers, they may now feel somewhat challenged by your increasing independence. Some relationships that worked well while you were ill may crumble once you become better, but some may just need to be renegotiated.

> Sam's partner was very supportive while he was ill. When he started getting better and began to do things for himself, he realized that she was not totally happy for him. She had obviously got something from being the person who did things for him and supported him. His independence was something of a threat. They had to work together at redefining their changed relationship.

## A new way of looking at life

It is possible that the pace of your life before you were ill was not sustainable and was more than you could have kept up indefinitely. If this was the case, it may be unwise to go back to that sort of lifestyle. Part of planning for the future should include thinking about why you pushed yourself so hard and accepting that repeating this pattern of behaviour could be a mistake. You may have to give up some ambitions and recognize that some of your previous activities are no longer possible. Pacing yourself more carefully to limit excessive demands may have to be part of your life for some time to come. The style of managing yourself we have talked about is likely to give you a real improvement, but it is not a guaranteed cure. You may need to be careful for a long time, but you do not have to think of this as second best. Being gentle with yourself could well be a life skill that will be of real benefit to you for the rest of your life.

It is possible to use this period of recovery in a constructive way. You have time to think about what you liked and did not like in your life before you were ill and, based on that, plan out a better future.

Getting better can be wonderful, but it can also pose a challenge. Accepting that there are problems can be the first stage in dealing with them. Lots of forward planning and information gathering will help. Voluntary or part-time work may be the route back into full employment. Relationships may have to be redefined. You may need to plan for a very different lifestyle from the one you had before you were ill, but different does *not* have to be worse.

# 30

# Summary of our self-help advice

We very much hope that you will try out the self-help techniques we have outlined in this section. Both research and increasing amounts of clinical experience have shown that they **can** result in an improvement in your condition. Over time they can make a great difference to your state of health and to your well-being. In the 15 years and more that we have been working with people with CFS/ME we have seen the benefits that can come from this approach. We do **not** say that these techniques will give you a cure, but they can give you the significant benefits of a decrease in symptoms and/or an increase in your level of functioning. You could try:

- To stabilize your rest–activity pattern, work towards improving your sleep, see that you eat healthily, and learn to relax and to manage pain. Aim for consistency.

- To manage your difficulties with memory and concentration.

- To do your best to stay as 'normal' as possible.

- To start the process of making very small and cautious increases in your activity, both physical and mental, once you have achieved stability and consistency.

- To look at 'what gets in the way of being sensible'.

- To do whatever is possible to improve your mood. If you suffer from anxiety, panic, or depression, use self-help techniques and/or accept professional help.

- To improve your skills in problem solving and communication.

- To work on improving relationships.

- To get the best you can from today while planning for the future.

♦ To think about the ways in which you will manage the changes that better health may bring. Use problem-solving techniques.

You do not need to put your life on hold waiting for some 'magic bullet' that will cure you. Maybe such a cure will be found, but it is not going to happen in the near future. In the meantime you can do a great deal to help yourself. You deserve a fulfilling life, not at some undetermined time in the future—but today.

# Section 3

# Special issues

# 31

# Thinking about therapies and therapists, both medical and complementary/ alternative

 Key points

♦ Trying out treatments (whether conventional medical or complementary/alternative ones) has advantages and disadvantages

♦ Before you decide on a treatment, think carefully about what you want from it

♦ You have a right to question a therapist before you agree to take part in treatment

♦ Monitor the effect of a treatment so that you can decide if it is worth you continuing with it

♦ Don't spend more time and money than you can afford

As we said in Chapter 8, there is no 'magic bullet' that will **cure** CFS/ME. However, most people would still like to believe that there must be a simple treatment out there that will at least help, and so they keep on looking. Making a choice between the enormous varieties of therapies available can be extremely difficult. We hope that what follows will help in making that choice.

# Therapies in general

We are not going to look here at any specific medical, complementary, or alternative treatment. Instead, we are going to talk about what we believe you should consider and the questions you should ask of both yourself and the therapist before embarking on any of them. Most of what we say can be applied to any treatment—conventional or complementary/alternative.

### Why do you want a treatment?

This may at first seem like a silly question to ask, but people do have very different reasons for seeking treatment. If you are clear about what you want to get from the treatment, it will help you to choose.

- Are you looking for a 'cure'? Do you believe that if you go on looking long enough you will eventually find one? The plain truth is that so far **nothing** has been found that will reliably **cure** CFS/ME. If that is your hope, we are afraid that you are probably heading for disappointment.

- Are you looking for something that will make you feel better generally, such as a reduction in symptoms?

- Are you looking for help with one or more specific symptoms?

- Are you looking for an increase in energy and an improvement in what you are able to do?

- Are you looking for ongoing support and encouragement?

- Are you unhappy with the treatment that your family doctor is offering you?

### Potential benefits of trying any treatment

- You may find it helpful.

- The idea that you are doing something to help yourself may give you a sense of control over the illness.

- Any reduction in symptoms, even if limited, will be welcome.

## Potential disadvantages of trying any treatment

- If you do improve, you may mistakenly give the credit to the therapy/ therapist rather than to what you are doing to help yourself or to the natural progress of the condition. This may reduce your feeling of being able to manage the illness yourself. You may then mistakenly conclude that continued improvement depends on continuing with the treatment.

- If the therapy does not do any good, having your expectations of cure or improvement disappointed may only add to your feelings of frustration and hopelessness.

- It may cost you a lot of money (which might be better spent on other things). Indeed we are concerned about the small minority of doctors and therapists who appear to take advantage of the desperate or the despairing.

- Treatments that rely on something given **to you** or something done **for you** by someone else can be a distraction from the things you can do **for yourself** that we discuss in this book.

- If you do not improve, some doctors and therapists may blame you— saying that you have not tried hard enough or persisted long enough. While this may sometimes be true, life with CFS/ME is tough enough without being unfairly blamed for not getting better.

- There is a small chance that some treatments will cause you harm.

## Looking at the evidence

In order to make the best choice of treatment you will have to consider what evidence there is for its effectiveness. In Chapter 1 we talked about the three levels of evidence—the anecdotal reports of other suffers, the opinion of therapists and doctors based on clinical experience, and evidence from sound clinical research, especially clinical trials. We also talked about the scepticism necessary when judging research. This scepticism and judgement of evidence is just as important when thinking about whether a treatment is right for you. You do not need to take anyone's word for it (even if they are a doctor).

You have a right to ask about the quality of the evidence for the treatment they are proposing.

## Questions you should ask the doctor or therapist (and yourself)

You have a right to question anyone offering you treatment before you agree to it. You do not need to be hesitant or embarrassed about doing this.

♦ What does this treatment offer you? Does it match with what you want from it? What evidence is there that this treatment has a good chance of doing this?

♦ Has there been any good-quality research, in particular good clinical trials, of the treatment? Is this still an experimental treatment?

♦ What exactly are the risks of side effects of this treatment?

♦ Is this treatment part of a research project? There can be advantages is taking part in research treatment as the care patients receive in trials is usually of a very high standard. You do not have to take part unless you choose to.

♦ How long is the treatment likely to take? Does the doctor/therapist insist on a minimum number of treatments and if so why?

♦ If you are paying for the treatment, how much is it going to cost in total (including tests, drugs, etc.)? Think about what you might have to give up to pay for it. Would you do better spending that money on something else that would make your life easier or give you pleasure? Some patients spend a great deal of money they can ill afford without being helped.

♦ What will be the cost to you of having the treatment in terms of your energy? Would you have to travel? Would the resulting fatigue outweigh the benefits?

♦ Does the doctor/therapist have experience of using this treatment in patients with CFS/ME? If so, in how many patients? What results has she or he had? Does he or she understand the problems you have?

♦ What training and qualifications does the therapist have? (It is not always easy to judge these for complementary and alternative therapists.)

♦ Does the therapist belong to a professional organization that monitors standards of treatment? (Again this is not always easy to judge for therapists giving complementary and alternative treatments.) Can that organization enforce standards? Is there a complaints procedure and does the therapist carry proper professional insurance?

◆ Will the therapist keep in touch with your usual doctor?

## Monitoring results

If after all this you decide to go ahead with a treatment, you do need to monitor your progress in order to decide if it is helping and whether to continue. This is why we suggest that you are clear about what you want from it. You may need to try more than just one single session or continue with a drug or supplement for a while before you can judge what it can offer you. The doctor/therapist should be able to advise you how long it will be before you should expect to see a result. If after taking this into account you are no better or worse, you have a right to stop. As a rough guide, if you cannot see any real benefit after 6–8 weeks, it might be better to stop. Do not let yourself be bullied into continuing if you do not want to. Give yourself a pause. You can then decide whether to continue or to try something else.

## Self-help is a treatment

We described self-help techniques earlier in this book. These are intended to help you to give your body the best chance of doing its own healing. They are just as much 'treatments' as any drug or alternative therapy. Do not be trapped into thinking 'If I'm only doing that, then I'm not doing the best for myself'. This applies just as much to the cognitive behaviour therapy (CBT) and graded exercise therapy (GET) which we discuss in the next chapter (which are very similar to self-help, but with expert back-up and support). Research evidence including repeated clinical trials has shown that, at the present time, these are the most effective treatments available. They are not a magic cure, but they can improve both your bodily state and your well-being, and help some people to recover. If you choose these treatments you will certainly be giving yourself a good chance of improvement. But—as with all treatments— ask questions and decide if they are the right treatments for you.

# Medical therapists and therapies

## The general practitioner

Your starting point is likely to be your own doctor. Happily, most people know and trust their general practitioner (GP). Most family doctors offer only ethical and reputable treatment. If you feel that your doctor does not understand your condition or is not giving you the best advice and treatment, do tell them of your concerns. If you really cannot sort things out, you may be able to see another doctor in the same practice who has more knowledge or interest in CFS/ME. As a last resort, you may decide to change your family doctor, but do remember that there are disadvantages as well as advantages of starting afresh with someone new.

## Specialist doctors

Your own doctor may refer you to a hospital specialist or special CFS/ME clinic. Hospital doctors are subject to the scrutiny of their colleagues and are answerable to professional regulatory bodies. These factors make it less likely that they will use treatments that are unethical or not firmly based on evidence. Furthermore, in the UK such treatment will probably be free of charge.

However, not all doctors treating CFS/ME are using evidence-based treatments. Do be particularly cautious about doctors who are not recommended by your own family doctor, who work on their own, or who are making money from selling treatments. Do make sure that you have satisfied yourself about the questions we suggested you ask before you agree to accept treatment from them. Do not spend more money than you can afford.

## 'Doctor shopping'

Once you have found a family doctor you are comfortable with and perhaps had an authoritative diagnosis from a medical specialist, you will probably do better to stick with that and concentrate on working to manage your condition. However, some people with CFS/ME feel that if they go on looking long enough and 'shop around' they will find the 'ideal doctor', someone who will truly understand both them and their condition and make them better. Such a search is likely to disappoint and can take up a great deal of time, energy, and money It will certainly be a distraction from working on ways of helping yourself.

## Conventional drug therapies

Probably the most important of these are the 'so-called' antidepressant drugs. Their use is described in Chapter 22. For some people they can help reverse the brain changes that are part of the illness. Other conventional therapies are largely symptom-relieving drugs. Used in a sensible way they can be useful, but you might want to try self-help techniques first.

### Experimental drug treatments

Some doctors, whether working in a hospital setting or on their own, use more experimental therapies. This may suit you and you might just be lucky enough to find something that really helps. On the other hand, you might find that many of these therapies do not help and may have some unpleasant or harmful effects. If you are being given a treatment of unproven value, this should ideally be as part of a properly evaluated research project. Participating in research can be a way to get better than standard treatment. But remember that you should understand fully what is involved and be asked to give your 'informed consent'.

### Non-drug treatments

A medical treatment does not have to involve taking a drug. There are also powerful 'non-drug' treatments or therapies. These include such things as CBT and GET (see Chapter 32). There are also a variety of medical therapists who can help with specific problems. For example, you could get help from physiotherapists for physical de-conditioning or specific muscle problems, or you could get psychological therapy from psychiatrists, psychologists, and counsellors for addressing emotional problems.

# Complementary/alternative therapists and therapies

These are treatments that lie outside conventional medicine. The distinction between 'complementary' and 'alternative' can be somewhat blurred. Complementary therapies are those to be used alongside conventional medicine. Indeed some doctors have trained in treatments such as homeopathy and acupuncture. Alternative therapies (as the name suggests) on the other hand are more likely to be suggested as an alternative to conventional treatment. As we said in Chapter 8, these therapies can range from things that your doctor might be happy to recommend, to some that are frankly bizarre and possibly dangerous.

### Potential advantages of complementary and alternative treatments

◆ Complementary and alternative therapies may appeal to you as more 'natural' than mainstream medicine.

◆ A complementary or alternative therapist may be able to give you more time than can a busy doctor. Just seeing someone who listens to your problems in a sympathetic way and who takes an interest in you as a person (not just as a 'case') can be helpful. Ongoing support can make managing any illness feel easier.

♦ You may prefer to choose a treatment for yourself rather than having your doctor decide for you.

## Potential disadvantages of complementary and alternative treatments

♦ In general, complementary and alternative therapists are subject to less regulation than doctors. There is therefore more opportunity for dubious treatment and unethical practice.

♦ Alternative therapies will usually cost you money. Be sure you can afford them.

♦ There is very little systematic research evidence for the effectiveness of most complementary and alternative therapies. This can make it very hard to judge how likely they are to help you.

♦ Some complementary or alternative practitioners suggest ideas about CFS/ME that have no scientific basis. They can be confusing and even fanciful. Whilst the suggestion that your illness has a simple cause (such as diet or dental fillings) may be initially encouraging, it is likely to be ultimately disappointing.

♦ You may find that your doctor feels less able to help you if you choose such therapies.

## A few warnings

Whilst some therapies can help with specific symptoms—for instance osteopathy or chiropractic can be useful treatments for some back problems—others have very little proven value or may even be potentially dangerous. We are concerned about the number of people with CFS/ME who have been advised to adopt very restricted diets or to take massive supplements of vitamins or minerals. Some therapists diagnose food sensitivities, allergies, or other problems by entirely unscientific methods.

You should be very cautious about any therapist who is not willing to make contact with your usual doctor. Be especially wary of suggestions that you must stop using conventional medicine. In particular do not stop any conventional medical treatment abruptly (for instance, antidepressant drugs) without first discussing this with your doctor. Also do note that some herbal remedies can conflict with medically prescribed drugs.

Many of the patients we have talked with report spending a great deal of time, energy, and money on alternative therapies (probably more than they could afford of all three) without getting any real benefit.

### Deciding to try a complementary/alternative treatment

Despite what we have said, you may have decided to try one of these therapies. In spite of the cautions we have highlighted, we are certainly not saying that you should not use them. Indeed there is *some* evidence that *some* therapies (such as homeopathy) can help *some* patients with *some* of their symptoms. Something like massage that you enjoy may make you feel a little better, at least for a while. All that we suggest is that you should think carefully about which ones you choose and consider the evidence for their effectiveness. Just because therapists tell you that something is effective, you do not have to believe them without them having given you good evidence. We have included a book in the further information list (Appendix 3) which could give you some guidance on choosing a therapy and a therapist.

You may already have felt under pressure from relatives, friends, or other people with CFS/ME to try a specific complementary or alternative therapy. People imply that if you are not trying these therapies then you are not really trying to get better. You may find that other people read something in the paper about the latest 'cure' and insist that you try it. **You** are the one with the illness and the one who has to take the treatment. **You** have a right to choose what you do—you do not need to give in to these pressures.

## Summary—where has all this got us?

Of course you would like there to be a treatment out there that will make you feel better. Trying some of them out may help you. Finding someone, whether a doctor, a complementary therapist, or an alternative therapist, who will look at you as a whole person (rather than just a collection of symptoms) and give you ongoing support can be very comforting. You can continue self-help techniques as well. However, if you are trying a mix of treatments, it can be hard to decide which one helps.

All we suggest is that you are cautious and selective about which treatments you choose. A search for the 'perfect' treatment that will solve all your problems is likely to be expensive, exhausting, and fruitless. It may also distract you from what you can do to help yourself.

Trying out treatments, whether medical or complementary/alternative therapies, can have advantages and disadvantages. Think first about what you are looking for from a treatment. You are likely to make a better choice if you look carefully at the evidence for the effectiveness of the treatment. You have a right to question the doctor or therapist before you agree to take part. You will also need to monitor the effect of the treatment in order to decide if it is worth continuing. Do not spend more money than you can really afford. Having a treatment does not mean that you should stop using self-help techniques—you can use both.

# 32

# Cognitive behaviour therapy, graded exercise therapy, and adaptive pacing therapy

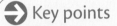 Key points

- Cognitive behaviour therapy (CBT) can help people suffering from psychological problems, depression, and anxiety, and also those suffering with physical symptoms such as chronic pain and those with CFS/ME

- Graded exercise (or more properly 'activity') therapy (GET) concentrates more on achieving very gradual increases in activity

- Adaptive pacing therapy (APT) concentrates on adapting to limitations and achieving a balance between rest and activity

These are the main treatments used by the National Health Service in the UK for CFS/ME. Cognitive behaviour therapy (CBT) and graded exercise therapy (GET) have the strongest evidence for effectiveness. Adaptive pacing therapy (APT) has been less well researched, but is supported by anecdote and by professional and patient experience.

## Cognitive behaviour therapy

CBT was originally developed over 30 years ago by an American psychiatrist Aaron Beck as a treatment for depression. Since then CBT has been adapted to treat many other conditions, both psychological and physical, including CFS/ME. There is a substantial body of research evidence that supports its effectiveness.

## The ideas behind CBT

CBT is based on the idea that the way you think about your illness (your cognitions) and the way you cope with it (your behaviour) influence its outcome. Your initial reactions to this idea might be:

1.  'Doesn't everyone think the same way about his or her illness?'

2.  'How can thinking and coping behaviour affect a physical illness?'

3.  'How could you change your thinking anyway?'

### Doesn't everyone think the same way about his or her illness?

People do not all think in the same way—look at the different ways they vote in an election! The more ambiguous the situation, the greater the variation in what people think about it.

Consider this example. You are in bed alone and you hear a noise downstairs. You do not know exactly what it is. What do you think? You might think it is an intruder—or you might decide it is just the cat. These are very different thoughts with very different effects on how you feel and how you behave. We probably do not need to emphasize to you that CFS/ME is an illness surrounded by misunderstanding and uncertainly—a situation likely to produce a variety of interpretations.

### How can thinking and coping behaviour affect a physical illness?

Thinking affects your mood, your behaviour, and your physiological (bodily) state. To continue our example, if you think that the noise is an intruder you are likely to be anxious (mood), jump out of bed (behaviour), and develop a faster heart rate (bodily state). These reactions will be the same whether the noise was an actual intruder or just the cat! It is your thoughts and beliefs that determine your reaction—not the reality. Persistently inaccurate thinking can lead to poor coping and to bad effects on emotion, behaviour, and bodily state. For instance, if a person worries constantly that things will go wrong, they will be chronically anxious, tend to avoid doing things, and be in a physiological state of tension and arousal.

These effects not only alter how you feel but can influence the course of illness. There is evidence that how people think about their illness affects how likely they are to recover. This may work by influencing what treatment they seek and how they cope (e.g. by getting fitter or by taking to bed). There may also be direct effects on the body—for example the functioning of the nervous and immune systems can be influenced by mood and coping behaviour.

### How could you change your thinking anyhow?

A central point of CBT is that you can choose what to think. You can look for evidence (e.g. by going downstairs and having a look and deciding that it was not an intruder but the cat knocking something over). The therapist helps you to choose what to think about your illness, not by a process of brain washing, but by support and guidance. You are the one who decides what to think.

## CBT for depression

People suffering from depression are typically low in mood. They also tend to have negative and inaccurate thoughts and beliefs about themselves, their circumstances, and their future. For example, they may think that they are a worthless person, in a hopeless predicament, and with no future. This type of distorted thinking was long believed to be simply a **result** of their depression. Beck's big idea was that this thinking could also be a **cause** of their depression and that by changing their thinking patients could get better.

CBT works by helping patients to think more accurately about themselves, their situation, and their future. This does not mean adopting equally inaccurate positive thinking, but rather getting evidence to find out the truth (in our example by going downstairs to see what is happening).

### What happens during CBT treatment for depression?

During the treatment sessions, the therapist helps the patients to be aware of their thinking and coping behaviour, and to consider alternatives. Between treatment sessions patients carry out 'homework' tasks. For instance, they may be set the task of keeping a record of negative thoughts about themselves ('I am a failure'). Once a person is aware of their thinking, they can be helped to look at more accurate and balanced alternative thoughts (e.g. 'Some things I have tried to do have failed, but others have succeeded. This does not make me a failure as a person.').

## CBT for anxiety and panic

Once CBT was an established treatment for depression, psychiatrists and psychologists went on to identify distorted thinking in patients with other problems such as anxiety, panic and phobias. For example, people who panic tend to 'catastrophize' their physical symptoms (a twinge of chest pain is interpreted as 'I'm having a heart attack and going to die'). They consequently pay great attention to how their body feels. A person with phobia tends to exaggerate the risk of normal behaviours (e.g. someone who fears flying may think 'There is a 90% chance that a plane will crash' and consequently avoid flying). New versions of CBT were then developed to help people with these problems.

## CBT for physical illnesses

In recent years, forms of CBT have been devised for people suffering from a wide range of physical conditions such as chronic pain, cancer, and the after effects of a heart attack. CBT can help people with these illnesses cope better. For instance, someone with chronic pain might be helped to return to previously enjoyed activities in spite of their pain.

## CBT for CFS/ME

### What it is not

Before we go on to talk about what CBT for CFS/ME **is**, it may help if we spell out what it **is not**:

◆ It is not another way of saying that CFS/ME is 'all in the mind'.

◆ It does not imply that a person with CFS/ME is failing to try.

◆ It does not imply that the only reason a person with CFS/ME stays ill is because of inaccurate beliefs about their illness.

◆ It is not 'a programme of ruthlessly increased exercise imposed on helpless CFS/ME victims'.

### What it is

CBT for CFS/ME is not really new. It was described by doctors treating neurasthenia more than 100 years ago; it was developed for CFS/ME more than 20 years ago and has been gradually refined. CBT is now offered in many centres. The therapists can be psychiatrists, psychologists, or trained nurse counsellors. We cannot emphasize enough that CBT should be a collaboration between the patient and the therapist—it is not **imposed** on them. Patients are assessed and treated as individuals. The aim is to help patients do more and feel better.

In Section 2 we outlined all the things that people with CFS/ME can do to help themselves. We know from experience that many people find it hard to do this on their own. It is easier to undertake and stick to such a programme with expert guidance and back-up. There will be bound to be times when you come up against problems and have doubts about what you are doing. Talking things through with the therapist can make quite a difference. It can also be helpful to have someone to whom you can report your successes, particularly if that person understands the difficulties you may have had to surmount to achieve that success.

### What happens during a course of CBT treatment?

The typical CBT course normally involves 10–16 hour-long sessions in which you talk to your therapist. They are usually scheduled weekly to begin with, but perhaps every fortnight later on. There may also be a follow-up session some months later to check how you are progressing. Patients are expected to do 'homework' between these sessions in which they try out new ways of coping.

### Does CBT work for people with CFS/ME?

Yes, it does seem to help. It is not a cure, but research including a number of clinical trials in different centres has shown that about two-thirds of patients who take part in such a programme are able to do more and feel better.

# Graded exercise therapy (GET)

GET is similar in many ways to CBT, but it concentrates more on changing coping behaviour rather than thinking. It might be better called graded activity therapy. The aim is to help the person with CFS/ME stabilize and then increase their **physical** activity (not just exercise). GET assumes that if the increases in activity are made gradually, the body will be able to tolerate being more active and that this will speed recovery.

In GET, the rate of increase is controlled by the patients—they will not be encouraged to move onto the next stage in the programme until they are ready. In the early stages, the increases in activity will be very small. Patients are likely to be asked to start with 5–15 minutes of gentle exercise. This amount can then be increased by 1 or 2 minutes at a time (depending on progress) up to a maximum of 30 minutes a day.

There is evidence from several clinical trials that GET can be helpful for some patients. It may well be that those it helps most are those suffering most from the effects of deconditioning. It may also be possible that at least some of the benefit comes from giving patients back the feeling that they can control their illness and help themselves.

## Adaptive pacing therapy (APT)

APT concentrates on coping behaviour. Like CBT and GET, the aim is to stabilize activity, Unlike CBT and GET there is no plan to increase activity. APT assumes that stabilizing activity allows natural recovery. The aim is to use pacing to avoid making symptoms worse—by balancing activity and rest and by not exceeding the available energy. The main strategies used in this pacing are establishing a stable and manageable baseline of activity, interspersing this with periods of proper rest. Although APT does not include gradual increases in activity, it is assumed that the person with CFS/ME will be able to make these as they begin to feel better.

Whilst the strategies used in APT are an important part of CBT and GET and have been found helpful by many patients, they have not yet been properly tested in a clinical trial.

## CBT, GET, and APT in CFS/ME

These are all treatments for CFS/ME that depend on the person changing how they cope, rather than on drugs. Each of these treatments has its exponents. There is most evidence for the effectiveness of CBT and also good evidence for GET. There is less evidence for APT, but anecdotally many patients have reported that they have found it helpful.

The PACE trial funded by the UK Medical Research Council is comparing these three treatments with basic specialist medical care alone. The findings of this trial will be available in 2010. You could look at their web site (www.pacetrial.org).

## 'So-called' CBT and GET

Unfortunately, therapies that are offered under the name of CBT, GET, and APT are not always as described here. Some health professionals have read only briefly about CBT and GET, and offer poor-quality treatment under those names. As with any other therapy, you have a right to question them about their training and experience before starting the therapy. We hope that you now have a much better idea of what real CBT and GET are like.

Cognitive behaviour therapy (CBT) can help people suffering from depression, anxiety, and panic. It can also help people suffering from physical illnesses including CFS/ME. It is not something imposed on patients and should be carried out with therapist and patient working together. It should be tailored to the individual patient's needs.

Graded exercise therapy (GET) is somewhat similar, but concentrates more on coping and increases in activity than on the person's thinking.

Adaptive pacing therapy (APT) focuses on balancing activity and rest. It has not yet been properly tested as a treatment on its own.

# 33

# Children and young people with CFS/ME

## ➲ Key points

◆ Good management is needed at an early stage

◆ With such management, the prognosis for a child is good, probably better than for an adult

◆ Most of the self-help techniques we described in Section 2 also apply to children

◆ It is stressful to have a child with CFS/ME. As his or her parents, you need to look after yourselves as well as the child

It is not only adults who can get CFS/ME. It is a sad fact that children and young people can suffer from it as well. Their symptoms are very similar to those experienced by adults, though they may not talk about being fatigued in quite the same way. Like adults, the onset of illness may be acute following a viral-type illness (such as glandular fever), or may be more gradual. As we have said before, the label CFS/ME probably covers more than one condition, so your child's illness may be very different from that of another child with the same diagnosis.

Obviously, an illness like this is intensely worrying and distressing for parents. Not knowing what to do for the best can add enormously to the load that parents have to bear. We hope that if you are a parent of a child with CFS/ME you will have read the earlier sections of this book and so feel a little more knowledgeable about what will help.

# Diagnosis

The way CFS/ME is diagnosed in children is much the same as that described for adults in Chapter 4. The major difference is that it is now agreed that it is appropriate to make a diagnosis in a child after 3 months of illness, rather than wait until they have been ill for 6 months.

The same sort of questions, examinations, and diagnostic tests are used to exclude other conditions that could produce similar symptoms. Some family doctors may call in other health professionals—a paediatrician or a child psychiatrist or psychologist for instance—to assist them in making the diagnosis and to exclude other conditions.

As with adults, these other conditions include emotional problems. In children, these include anxiety about going to school (school phobia), anorexia nervosa, and depression. (Yes, children can suffer from depression.) As a parent you may feel that your child's illness could not possibly be emotional. However, it is worth being open to the possibility that he or she has one of these conditions, because this may lead to effective treatment.

Do not be too alarmed if your child is given a diagnosis of CFS/ME. In our experience, the cases that have been given attention in the newspapers and on television are unusually severe. You really do have grounds for reasonable optimism.

# Prognosis

Studies that have examined the outcome of children who have received a diagnosis of CFS/ME show that, in general, the outlook is good for children and certainly better than for adults. This seems to be especially true if the children and their families have received good advice and help early in the illness. Although recovery may take some time, the majority of children are much improved by 2 years after onset. Even if your child has been ill for a longer time than this, effective rehabilitation is possible. Most children do recover and go on to lead normal lives.

# Getting help

The help that parents and children get from their general practitioners and other health professionals is important in achieving a good outcome for a child with CFS/ME. That is why it is so important to establish a positive working relationship with them. You might want to refer to Chapter 25 on how to get the best from your doctor.

You may feel that your family doctor does not fully understand your child's problems. If you have concerns about this, express them calmly and clearly. If you are still unhappy, see if there is another doctor in the practice who has greater interest and expertise in childhood CFS/ME. If all else fails, you might want to change doctors, but do be aware that this means starting again with somebody new.

You may also feel that if only you could find the right specialist your child could be made better. In reality, most paediatricians are familiar with CFS/ME, and there is probably little to be gained from seeking second and further opinions. If you do decide to seek further opinions, beware of the negative effect that multiple opinions and fragmented care can have on your child.

Help may come not only from the doctor, but also from the other people who may become involved in the care of an ill child—teachers, educational psychologists, educational authorities, social services, etc. Do use your experience as a parent to keep them informed of your child's difficulties, needs, and progress. Teachers or doctors may only see the child for a short time and not be aware of some of the difficulties. For instance, teachers may not be aware that your child has problems with memory and concentration, or that mental activity can be as tiring as physical.

## Self-help—achieving a balance

So what can parents do to give their child the best chance of recovery? Everything we have said about helping yourself in Section 2 applies just as much to children and young people as it does to adults. The key points are to ensure that the diagnosis is correct, to treat problems such as depression, to establish a manageable daily routine, and then to work towards a gradual return to normal activity. However, because children are much more dependent on the adults around them, are growing and developing, and are still in education, they have additional needs. It is important for the parents themselves to work toward a balance between pushing children and treating them as 'poor darlings' who have to have everything done for them.

## Balancing the day

Children with CFS/ME often lose the usual daily routine and may need guidance and help to structure their day. The overall aim is to establish a manageable and regular routine of sleeping, eating, and activity.

## Sleeping

It is very important to maintain or re-establish a regular pattern of sleep. If children have slept badly, it can be very tempting to let them sleep on later and later into the morning. It is much better to stick to a regular, normal waking time. If this is not done, the child can end up sleeping most of the day and being awake most of the night. Our advice on improving sleep in Chapter 15 applies to children as well as adults. As with adults, a small dose of a sedative antidepressant can help with sleep problems, though this is something you would need to discuss with your child's doctor.

## Eating and diet

Regular meal times are important. Anything that keeps a normal rhythm going during the day will be helpful. Try to stick to normal meal times (although it may suit some children better to include small healthy snacks at set times between meals). Allowing 'grazing' just when a child feels like eating is probably not a good idea.

Growing children need good food. Their meals should include all the food groups (as discussed in Chapter 16). Whatever you may read or hear, most children do not need special diets. However, calcium is essential for the development of strong bones, so if it has really been **proved** that a child is intolerant of milk products, supplements of calcium may be needed. Discuss this with your doctor.

## Balancing activity with rest and relaxation

Children need both rest and activity for good health. This balance is likely to have been upset by the illness. It is best to begin by establishing a pattern of rest and activity that your child can manage on a daily basis. Time-limited periods of activity (both physical and mental) alternated with good-quality rest, spread evenly through the day, are probably best. The length of the initial periods of activity will obviously depend on just how much an individual child can manage. The aim is to achieve a programme which does not increase symptoms too much and which can be managed every day in a consistent way. Read Chapter 12 on 'Balancing rest and activity'.

Prolonged bed rest in particular is to be avoided. It has an effect on the body called deconditioning, which causes weak muscles and other problems (as we discussed in Chapter 14). Complete bed rest quickly produces deconditioning, which is to be avoided. Whilst some time in bed may be necessary for a number of days after an acute illness, this rest period should be kept brief. It has been plausibly argued that **some** of the symptoms that children with CFS/ME experience may in fact be the result of too much time in bed, resulting in de-conditioning.

The child may need to be encouraged to get out of bed and walk, even if it is only for a few steps at intervals during the day. Later on, longer distances and more vigorous exercise should be possible. Exercise periods should be planned so that they are within the child's current capacity and end before the child becomes too tired. The lengths of these periods of activity will obviously depend initially on just how much an individual child can manage. As with adults, pacing is vital—stopping before fatigue becomes excessive.

Good-quality rest is also important. The best rest comes when the child is really relaxed both in body and in mind (see Chapter 13). Even quite young children can be taught how to relax (one of the authors taught her own young children). If you can teach children how to relax, you will be giving them a tool that will be useful to them for the rest of their lives.

# Rehabilitation

Once such a stable routine is established, rehabilitation can begin. The lengths of the periods of activity (both physical and mental) can then be increased very gradually. The pace of increase should be within the child's capacity and manageable. A physiotherapist may be able to help here.

# Balancing appropriate discipline and too much control

Even quite small children need to feel that they have some control over themselves and their lives. It is not always easy to find the right balance between the degree of discipline that every child needs and allowing your child choices. This is especially so when that child is ill. This may be especially hard for parents who experienced similar difficulties when they were children. This ability to identify with your child can be both an advantage and a disadvantage. It is an advantage in helping you understand your child and how they might be feeling. It can, however, be a disadvantage when it comes to imposing necessary discipline, for example about attending school.

Striking a balance can be difficult. Nevertheless, it is important to your child's recovery and worth working at. It is also an area where the observations of a more 'objective' professional may often be helpful.

# Social contact

This is a vital need for a child's development, so it is important to explore ways in which social contact can be kept up. For example, a child with CFS/ME will almost certainly be able to cope with **short** visits from friends. You can help by making it easy and pleasant for visitors (a reputation for providing wonderful cakes helps!). If your child cannot cope with even short visits, then you could explore other methods—telephone calls (though you may need to ration the time spent on the phone), letters, or postcards to friends. These days, many children can use computers so e-mail could be another way of making contact, but there again you might need to limit time spent on the computer. A small kitchen timer can be useful to limit the time spent on an activity.

# Education

Obviously, an illness like this can have a major effect on a child's education. There are no hard and fast rules on how to deal with this—each child must be assessed as an individual. It is a good idea to talk to teachers early on so that they can help with how to keep the child's education going. A return to school is the ultimate aim, even if only part-time at first.

When the time comes to return to school, this is best planned well in advance. Doing too much too soon can lead to a setback and to loss of confidence. A part-time return—a few lessons a week in school—can help to maintain a normal life and to keep up social contact. Academic education and exams can wait for a while. It is surprising how quickly children can catch up once they recover. Even though a child is eager to return to school, absence may lead to anxiety about coping when he or she goes back. It can be helpful to bring this out into the open and discuss it. If your child does talk about problems about returning to school, you can help him or her to overcome these using a technique called 'problem solving', which is described in Chapter 24. (We have found that children as young as 5 years old can understand and use problem solving.)

In some cases when going to school does not seem possible, home tuition may be considered. This has advantages in helping the child who is too ill to keep up with school, but has the major disadvantage of not providing the normal school social environment. It is best, therefore, only used for a limited period.

# Emotions and emotional problems

Adults with CFS/ME can have emotional problems as part of the illness. Children are no different. Children may feel frightened, resentful, grief, anxious, and angry. They may already be facing the challenges of adolescence and demands of school, which are further complicated by the illness. They may find it hard to express these feelings. Furthermore, the expression of their distress may get all mixed up with feeling physically unwell.

It will help them if they can talk about their predicament and how they feel. They may find it easier to talk freely to someone outside the immediate family, so contact with a nurse, counsellor, or child psychologist can be useful. Openness within the family is also important. Some parents feel that they should try to maintain a calm and optimistic manner at all times so as 'not to upset' the child. However, this can lead to children with CFS/ME believing that their feelings (which may be neither calm nor optimistic) are not important or that it is bad to express them. This only adds to their problems.

If depression or anxiety is a block to progress, this is best treated. As with adults, both psychological help and medication for depression may have an important role in helping them recover.

## Self-esteem

Any illness can undermine a child's sense of self-esteem. You can help here— setting small achievable targets and giving praise for even small successes will be important.

Teenagers in particular care about their appearance. You may be able to help them with that. (Could you arrange for a visiting hairdresser or get a supply of suitable mail order catalogues from which to choose new clothes?)

## Families

It is difficult and distressing when a child has a prolonged illness, especially a poorly understood one. Inevitably, there is likely to be an effect on the whole family. Parents suffer distress, worry, and fear for the future, and sometimes guilt if the child does not improve. The strain of dealing with a child with CFS/ME can also put stress on the parents' own relationship, particularly if they hold differing views on how the child should be managed. Relatives can sometimes interfere and cause problems. It will be best for the child if you can talk about the problems, both between yourselves and perhaps also with professionals who can help.

Other children in the family may also feel the effects of their sibling's illness. They may feel anxious about their brother or sister, while at the same time feeling resentment at the increased attention that the parents are giving to that child—perhaps feeling that they themselves are being neglected. This can disturb the balance of relationships to the extent that the whole family needs help—not just the child that is ill.

## Looking after yourself

Being a parent of a child with CFS/ME is a strain. You cannot keep going all day every day without it taking its toll. This is especially true if your child's difficulty awakens unhappy memories from your own childhood, if you feel it is reflecting badly on your ability as a parent, or if you feel professionals are not helping. You need to look after yourself as well as your child. Do not feel guilty if, at times, you feel resentful at the way your child's illness has changed your life. Try to build in breaks for yourself, even if it is only just for an hour or two each day. That will ease the burden on you a little and help you to stand back from your problems for a while. You might even want to get some support from a counsellor for yourself. Your health and emotional well-being are vital to your child; look after them.

Good management at an early stage will give a child with CFS/ME the best chance of improvement and ultimate recovery. This is likely to involve:

* achieving a balance in their daily life and planning rehabilitation

* re-establishing regular sleep

* regular eating and a balanced diet

* planning periods of physical and mental activity balanced with good-quality rest

* encouraging appropriate levels of exercise that are very gradually increased

* keeping schooling and social contact going and working toward a full return

* dealing positively with emotional problems.

Remember, the welfare of the whole family needs to be looked after as well as that of the child who is ill. Look after yourself if you are a parent and use all the help you can get.

# Appendix 1

# Medical glossary

If you or a family member suffers from CFS/ME, it is likely that you may meet with some medical terms you do not understand, perhaps things you hear from your doctor or that you read in medical reports, textbooks, or research papers. We are well aware that doctors are inclined to use 'doctor speak' and forget that their audience may not understand some of their language. Sometimes a word used medically has a rather different meaning from when it is used in ordinary speech. The following is a brief list of some of the more commonly used terms, with definitions taken mostly from the *Oxford Concise Medical Dictionary*.

**acute** describing a disease of rapid onset, severe symptoms, and brief duration (compare this with *chronic*)

**adrenal glands** two endocrine glands situated on top of the kidneys. They produce hormones including adrenaline (epinephrine) and cortisol

**adrenaline** (epinephrine) a hormone which prepares the body for 'fight, flight, orfreeze' and has widespread effects on circulation, the muscles, and sugar metabolism

**antidepressants** drugs that have proven benefit in people with depressive disorder. They also have wider actions on pain, sleep, appetite, and energy. 'Antidepressant' is a misleading name for these 'brain tonics'

**arthralgia** pain in a joint

**autonomic nervous system** the part of the nervous system responsible for the control of bodily functions that are not consciously directed, such as regular beating of the heart, intestinal movements, sweating, salivation, etc.

**biopsy** the removal of a small piece of living tissue for microscopic examination

**biopsychosocial** an approach that takes into account biological, psychological, and social factors

**cerebral** of the brain

**chronic** describing an illness that has gone on for a long time. It does not imply anything about its severity (compare this with *acute*)

**circadian rhythms** regular cyclic changes within the period of about a day which govern many vital functions such as sleep, feeding, metabolism, and the secretion of many hormones

**coeliac disease** a condition in which the small intestine fails to digest and absorb food. It is due to a sensitivity of the intestinal lining to a protein contained in gluten (found in wheat, barley, and rye)

**cognitive function** the mental processes involved in memory, concentration, and attention

**cohort** a group of people chosen for a research project

**cortisol** a hormone produced and released by the adrenal glands. It is important for the normal response to any stress or infection

**cryptic** something concealed, or of unknown origin

**cytokines** chemicals produced by cells of the immune system

**debility** weakness or feebleness

**endocrine system** glands that manufacture hormones and secrete them directly into the bloodstream. They include the pituitary, thyroid, parathyroid, and adrenal glands, as well as the ovaries and testes

**endogenous** arising within or derived from the body

**enterovirus** any virus that enters the body through the gastrointestinal tract and multiplies there

**enzyme** a type of protein that is essential for normal functioning and development of bodily systems

**epidemiology** the study of the occurrence, pattern, and control of diseases in populations

**exogenous** the opposite of endogenous—originating outside of the body

**fasciculation** muscle twitching, seen as a flicker of movement under the skin

**heterogeneous** not all the same, composed of different types

**hormone** a substance that is produced in one part of the body, passes into the bloodstream, and is carried to other organs or tissues where it affects their functioning

**HPA (hypothalamic–pituitary–adrenal) axis** the systems connecting and including the hypothalamus, the pituitary gland, and the adrenal glands. It is central to the response to stress

**hyper-** a prefix meaning either over (as in physically above) or higher than normal

**hypersomnia** sleeping more than normal

**hypertension** blood pressure higher than normal

**hypo-** a prefix meaning underneath or less than normal

**hypoglycaemia** a deficiency of glucose in the bloodstream causing muscular weakness and incoordination, mental confusion, and sweating

**hypoperfusion** blood flow less than normal

**hypotension** blood pressure lower than normal

**hypothalamus** a region of the brain below the thalamus. It controls the pituitary gland which lies below it and regulates body temperature, thirst, hunger and eating, water balance, and sexual function

**iatrogenic** refers to a condition which has resulted from medical treatment, as either an unforeseen or inevitable side effect

**idiopathic** describing a condition the cause of which is unknown

**immune system** the organs responsible for immunity

**immunity** the body's ability to resist infection

**libido** sexual interest and drive

**magnetic resonance imaging (MRI)** a method of obtaining high-quality pictures of the inside of the body using high-powered magnets rather than X-rays

**medically unexplained** describing a condition or set of symptoms whose cause cannot be identified by standard medical tests. This does not mean that no cause exists, merely that no cause has been identified

**melatonin** a hormone produced by the pineal gland that helps synchronize the body to the 24-hour night and day rhythm (circadian rhythm)

**mental** relating to or affecting the mind

**multiple sclerosis (MS)** a chronic relapsing disease of the nervous system. The myelin sheaths surrounding nerves in the brain and spinal cord are damaged, affecting the function of the nerves involved

**myalgia** pain in the muscles

**neuroendocrine** the system of dual control of certain activities of the body by means of both nerves and circulating hormones

**neurotransmitter** a chemical substance released from nerve endings to transmit impulses to other nerves—the chemical messengers in the brain

**osteoporosis** loss of bony tissue, resulting in bones that are brittle and liable to fracture. A diet with adequate calcium, exercise, and hormone replacement therapy for post-menopausal women can help prevent it

**palpitation** an awareness of an irregularity in the heartbeat

**paraesthesia** numbness or tingling sensations sometimes called pins and needles

**pharmaceutical** relating to drugs used medically

**pituitary gland** the master endocrine gland responsible for producing a range of hormones, some of which regulate the secretion of hormones from other glands

**placebo** a medicine or treatment that is ineffective but may help to relieve a condition because the patient has faith in its powers. New drugs are tested against placebos in clinical trials

**plasma** the straw-coloured fluid in which the blood cells are suspended

**psychiatric** relating to psychiatry

**psychiatry** a branch of medicine that treats patients whose condition are, or were previously thought to be, 'mental'. It is increasingly apparent that these are disturbances of brain function. For example, patients with depression have altered levels of certain neurotransmitters

**psychological** relating to psychology

**psychology** the science and study of the mind, emotion, behaviour, and mental processes

**RNA (ribonucleic acid)** a chemical found in cells that helps to make proteins

**somatic** relating to the body rather than the mind

**somatization** refers to a process whereby emotional distress produces physical complaints

**somatization disorder** a chronic condition characterized by multiple recurrent physical symptoms that are unexplained by identifiable disease and often attributed to somatization

**stress** anything that leads to a stress response in the person exposed to it. Stress may be physical (such as noise), psychological (such as worry about work), or social (such as personal attacks). Chronic stress may lead to the development of illnesses such as depression and CFS/ME

**T-cells (T-lymphocytes)** white blood cells which are part of the immune system

**thyroid gland** a large endocrine gland situated in the base of the neck. It is concerned with the regulation of the metabolic rate by the secretion of thyroid hormone

**virology** the study and science of viruses

# Appendix 2

# Keeping a diary

## When you start a pacing programme

Keeping an activity diary for 2 or 3 weeks can be a good start to working out a 'pacing programme'. The information from it often shows you how the way that you are managing your day affects how you are feeling. The simplest way is to use a notebook with one page per day. It is a good idea to carry it round with you and enter things as they happen—if you wait till the end of the day to write it up you may well forget quite a lot.

The basic idea is to keep a record of all of your activities (both physical and mental), how long they took, and how you are feeling both physically and emotionally.

You need four columns:

1. *Time*—when you started an activity and when you stopped, so you can know how long you continued.

2. *Activity*—both physical and mental activities.

3. *How you are feeling physically*—your level of fatigue, malaise, pain, etc.

4. *How you are feeling emotionally*—happy or sad, satisfied, or frustrated, etc.

After a while you will probably be able to spot some patterns such as the 'roller coaster'. For instance, if you record a day during which you mostly felt very unwell physically and rather low emotionally, you may well notice that that day came after one or more days when you regularly pushed yourself to exhaustion. It is very typical of CFS/ME that the bad effects of getting too tired do not show up until the next day or even the day after that. You may also notice how getting exhausted can leave you feeling in very low spirits.

This sort of diary keeping will help give you some data about how long you can keep up various activities without getting too exhausted—you will have a much better idea of what the right 'bite size' is for you at the moment.

You will also get some data to help you spread out your activities throughout the day and throughout the week. It is likely that you will be surprised to find that some activities that you did not think of as particularly strenuous do tire you more than you realized. You may then decide that these need to be rationed for the time being.

We do not suggest that you should go on keeping such a diary for very long, in fact we think that it can be counter-productive. The process can be tedious and it may make you concentrate too much on 'symptom scanning' and so notice your symptoms much more. However, it can be very helpful at the beginning of your 'pacing programme'. You may find that going back to it for a week or two is useful if you find yourself getting a bit 'off course' in your pacing.

## What gets in the way of being sensible?

In Chapter 20 we talked about catching your thoughts just as you are about to start an activity or when you decide to continue it. This can often give you far greater insight into why you are doing things. Just trying to remember these thoughts is often not very successful. It is often better to carry a small notebook in your pocket and write your thoughts down as they happen. After a while you will probably be able to spot the things that push you into doing too much or too little.

## Achievements and happiness diary

It can often be very helpful to keep a diary in which you record only your moments of pleasure, satisfaction, or mastery. Recording what you are 'getting right' can make it easier to identify the moments when you are achieving a good balance between rest and activity, as well as the sort of things that improve your quality of life. Building on successes is always a good idea.

Often when people are unwell they tend to concentrate more on what is wrong with their lives than what is right. They tend to forget the good times because the bad times are so much more memorable. Keeping a diary that focuses on the good times does help keep things in perspective.

## Diary keeping does not have to be a way of life

Some people do find that it helps them to manage themselves better if they make diary keeping a permanent feature of their lives, but it is certainly not essential. On the whole we have found that keeping specific diaries (such as the ones we have suggested) at definite stages of your self-help programme can be useful, but focusing too much on symptoms can be counter-productive. If you find that you are letting your pacing slip, then it may be helpful to return to keeping an activity diary for a while. If you find yourself in low spirits and think that nothing good ever happens to you, then going back to keeping a satisfaction diary can help remind you that you do still have good moments. Recording achievements can boost your sense of self-esteem.

You are a unique person and can work out what works for you. As always in this illness, **you** are the person in control and can choose what you do. However, what we do **not** recommend is keeping the sort of diary that concentrates on 'doom and gloom'. That is likely to lower your spirits in a way that will not do you any good at all.

# Appendix 3
# Further information

Inevitably, we have not been able to cover everything about CFS/ME in a book of this length. We make some suggestions here of sources of further information.

## Research papers

Here is a selection of papers, published in reputable journals, about some of the topics we have discussed throughout the book. We have chosen these both to give you more information about research and to demonstrate that what we have said about CFS/ME is backed up by proper research.

### CDC (Centers for Disease Control) international case definition

Fukada, K., Straus, S.E., Hickie, I.B., Sharpe, M., Dobbins, J.G., and Komaroff, A.L. (1994) Chronic fatigue syndrome: a comprehensive approach to its definition and management. *Annals of Internal Medicine*, **121**, 953–9.

### Oxford case definition

Sharpe, M., Archard, L.C., Banatvala, J.E., Borysiewicz, L.K., Clare, A.W., David, A., *et al.* (1991) A report—chronic fatigue syndrome: guidelines for research. *Journal of the Royal Society of Medicine*, **84**, 118–21.

### Canadian case definition

Carruthers, B.M., Jain, A.K., De Meirleir, K.L., Peterson, D.L., Klimas, N.G., Lerner, A.M., *et al.* (2003) Myalgic encephalomyelitis/chronic fatigue syndrome: clinical working case definition, diagnostic and treatment protocols. *Journal of Chronic Fatigue Syndrome*, **11**, 7–116.

## Major recent reviews in leading journals

Prins, J.B., Van der Meer, J.W., and Bleijenberg, G. (2006) Chronic fatigue syndrome. *Lancet*, **367**, 221–355.

Afari, N., and Buchwald, D. (2003) Chronic fatigue syndrome: a review. *American Journal of Psychiatry*, **160**, 221–36.

## Overlap between CFS and related conditions

Wessely, S., Nimnuan, C., and Sharpe, M. (1999) Functional somatic syndromes: one condition or many? *Lancet*, **354**, 936–39.

## Chronic Lyme disease

Feder, H.M. Jr, Johnson, B.J., O'Connell, S., Shapiro, E.D., Steere, A.C., Wormser, G.P. for the Ad Hoc International Lyme Disease Group (2007) A critical appraisal of 'chronic Lyme disease'. *New England Journal of Medicine*, **357**, 1422–30.

# Using the Internet

More and more people are turning to the Internet as a source of information about many things including their illness. It is not necessary to own a computer to do this—many public libraries have computer facilities that can be used by the public and there are Internet cafes in most high streets where you can 'surf the net' for a modest fee.

The national patient support groups all have their own websites. Another source of information and support on the Internet is the discussion lists (support groups) and chat rooms for CFS/ME or CFIDS. We would urge you, however, to take into account everything we have said about a suitable level of scepticism about what you read. There are a vast amount of postings ranging from the good to the very unreliable.

Two things may help you in evaluating information.

First, the DISCERN instrument (see www.discern.org.uk/discern_instrument). This is a series of 15 questions you should ask yourself as you read through anything about treatment choices:

1. Are the aims clear?
2. Does it achieve its aims?
3. Is it relevant?

4. Is it clear what sources of information were used to compile the publication (other than the author or producer)?

5. Is it clear when the information used or reported in the publication was produced?

6. Is it balanced and unbiased?

7. Does it provide details of additional sources of support and information?

8. Does it refer to areas of uncertainty?

9. Does it describe how each treatment works?

10. Does it describe the benefits of each treatment?

11. Does it describe the risks of each treatment?

12. Does it describe what would happen if no treatment is used?

13. Does it describe how the treatment choices affect overall quality of life?

14. Is it clear that there may more than one possible treatment choice?

15. Does it provide support for shared decision making?

You need to rate the answers on a scale from 1 to 5. If you can, it is worth looking at the web site which gives guidance on answering. You will find more details about DISCERN in our book *Living with a long-term illness: the facts*.

Second, *The Patient's Internet Handbook* by Robert Kiley and Elizabeth Graham and published by the Royal Society of Medicine Press, 2001. This is an invaluable book if you want to look for medical information on the Internet.

## Useful web sites

*The NICE Guidelines on CFS/ME*

◆ **www.nice.org.uk/guidance/index/.jsp?action=byID&o=11824**

*Drugs*

◆ **www.bnf.org** is the website of the British National Formulary

◆ **www.intelihealth.com** is the website of the US Pharmacopoeia

*Doctors*

◆ **www.pocketdoctor.co.uk** gives examples of questions to ask your doctor in a variety of circumstances

◆ **www.patients-association.com** has a good section on dealing with doctors

*Pain*

◆ **www.inputpainunit.net** has interesting information about self-management techniques for pain, a good reading list, and some useful links to other sites

*Support groups for CFS/ME*

◆ Action for ME—**www.afme.org.uk**

◆ The ME Association—**www.meassociation.org.uk**

◆ The CFIDS Association—**www.cfids.org**

# Books

We have picked out some books that you might find helpful if you want to find out more about various aspects of CFS/ME or about ways in which you can help yourself. It may seem like a long list, but we are certainly not suggesting that you should read them all! Your local library may be able to obtain some of these for you to borrow, or you could buy second-hand copies from online bookshops.

## About CFS/ME

*Chronic Fatigue and its Syndromes.* Simon Wessely, Matthew Hotopf, and Michael Sharpe. Oxford University Press, 1999—a readable but large textbook, partly written by one of us. Intended for doctors, this book takes a comprehensive approach to the whole question of chronic fatigue as well as CFS/ME. ISBN 0192621815.

*Chronic Fatigue Syndrome: An Integrative Approach to Evaluation and Treatment.* Edited by Mark A. Demitrack and Susan E. Abbey. The Guilford Press, 1996—another textbook for doctors, but easier to read than some. ISBN 1572304995.

## Looking after yourself

*Back in Ten Minutes.* Mary Rintoul and Bernard West. Penguin, 1995—a very practical book about ways to avoid back problems. It contains really clear illustrations of suggested exercises. ISBN 0140234829.

*The New Complete New Guide to Massage.* Susan Mumford. Hamlyn, 2006—will give you ideas about massage you can do yourself or train someone else to do. ISBN 060615634.

*Coping Successfully with Pain.* Nevil Shone. Sheldon Press, 2002—techniques for self-help with pain. ISBN 0859698504.

*The Which? Guide to Complementary Medicine.* Barbara Rowlands. Which? Books, 2002—a good guide to complementary and alternative therapies, with sensible suggestions about choosing a therapist. ISBN 0852028938.

*Living with a Long-term Illness: The Facts.* Frankie Campling and Michael Sharpe. Oxford University Press, 2006—our second book about managing illness. It covers a lot of the same subjects as this one, but goes into greater detail. ISBN 0198538835.

*Managing More with Less.* Joanna Howard. Butterworth Heineman, 1997—although this book is aimed at people at work, most of what it says can be applied to normal life. ISBN 075063698X.

## Help with your emotions

*Manage Your Mind.* Gillian Butler and Tony Hope. Oxford University Press, 2007—one of the best self-help books, covering a wide range of subjects. It is written in a very clear way and is full of common sense. It has good chapters on dealing with worry and anxiety, problem solving, relationships, and communication. ISBN 0198527721.

*Overcoming Anxiety.* Helen Kennerley. Robinson, 1998—self-help techniques for dealing with anxiety. ISBN 1854874225.

*Panic Attacks.* Christine Inghams. Thorsons, 2000—self-help techniques for dealing with panic. ISBN 0007706904.

*Overcoming Depression.* Paul Gilbert. Robinson, 2000—self-help techniques for dealing with depression. ISBN 1841191256.

*Mind Over Mood.* Dennis Greenberger and Christine Padesky. The Guilford Press, 1995—one of the best books about cognitive behaviour therapy self-help techniques for dealing with anxiety, panic, and depression. ISBN 0898621283.

*The Which? Guide to Counselling and Therapy.* Mike Brookes and Shamil Wanigaratne. Which? Books, 2003—a helpful book which explains what is involved in counselling and different psychotherapies, as well as giving sensible advice on choosing a therapist. ISBN 0852029233.

*Getting to Yes: The Secret to Successful Negotiation.* Roger Fisher and William Ury. Random House Business Books, 2003—a good book if you want to learn more about negotiation and communication styles. ISBN 1844131467.

## Children and young people

*Somebody Help ME.* Jill Moss. Sunbow Books, 1995—a sensible self-help guide for young sufferers. ISBN 0952578301.

*A Parent's Guide to CFIDS—How to be an Advocate for Your Child with Chronic Fatigue Immune Dysfunction Syndrome.* David Bell, Mary Robinson, Jean

Pollard, Tom Robinson, and Bonnie Floyd. Haworth Medical Press, 1999—an American guide for parents, particularly looking at education. ISBN 0201407973.

## Relaxation

You may decide that you need help in learning how to relax. Helpful tapes and literature can be obtained by writing to:

Oxford Cognitive Therapy Centre
Warneford Hospital
Oxford OX3 7JX, UK

Or:

Talking Life (**www.talkinglife.co.uk**) at PO Box 1, Wirral, CH47 7DD, UK. This is a good source of tapes and CDs on a variety of subjects. We can thoroughly recommend their relaxation kit as well as some others. It could be worth getting their catalogue.

# Index